THE EIGHT BROCADES

Robert Poyton

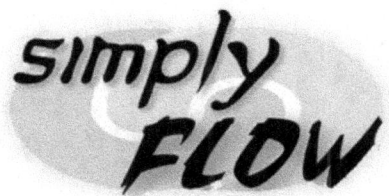

Copyright@ 2019 R Poyton

All rights reserved

The moral right of the author has been asserted

No part of this book may be reproduced in any form or by any electronic or mechanical means including information storage and retrieval systems, without permission in writing from the author. The only exception is by a reviewer, who may quote short excerpts in a review.

The author and publisher take no responsibility for any illness or injury resulting from practicing the exercises described in this book. Always consult your Doctor prior to training or if you have any medical issues.

Published by Cutting Edge

ISBN: 978-1-64606-427-4

"The clouds above us join and separate,

The breeze in the courtyard leaves and returns.

Life is like that, so why not relax?

Who can stop us from celebrating?"

— Lu Yu

TITLES IN THE SIMPLY FLOW SERIES

Fitness Over 40

The Human Gym

Ten Minute Tai Chi

The Eight Brocades

Fitness for Riders

Weight Training for Health

The Back Book

Stress Management

CONTENTS

CHAPTER ONE: INTRODUCTION
Introduction 9
How to use this book 11
Qigong 12
Traditional Chinese Medicine 16

CHAPTER TWO: FUNDAMENTALS
The Four Pillars 23
Stance 31
Zhan Zhuang 32
Speed 34
Open and Close 35
Acupuncture Points 37
Silk Reeling 40
Grounding 43

CHAPTER THREE: THE EIGHT BROCADES
The Eight Brocades 45
Opening 46
Two Hands Hold Up Heavens ... 48
Pulling Bow to Shoot 50
Separating Heaven and Earth ... 52
Turn and Gaze at the Moon ... 54
Sway Head and Shake the Tail ... 56
Two Hands Hold the Feet 58
Clench the Fists 60
Bouncing on the Toes 62
Closing and Grounding 64

CHAPTER FOUR: VARIATIONS
Variations 67
Separating with Turn 68
Separating to the Sides 70
Sway Head and Shake the Tail 72
Two Hands Hold the Feet 74
Seated Eight Brocades 76

CHAPTER FIVE: PRACTICE
Practice 79

APPENDIX ONE
The Eight Brocade Verses 84

APPENDIX TWO
Meridian Charts 86

APPENDIX THREE
Contact Details 95

左右開弓似射鵰

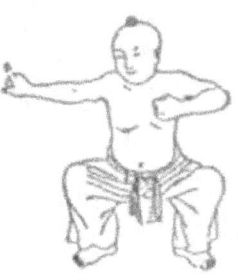

CHAPTER ONE
INTRODUCTION

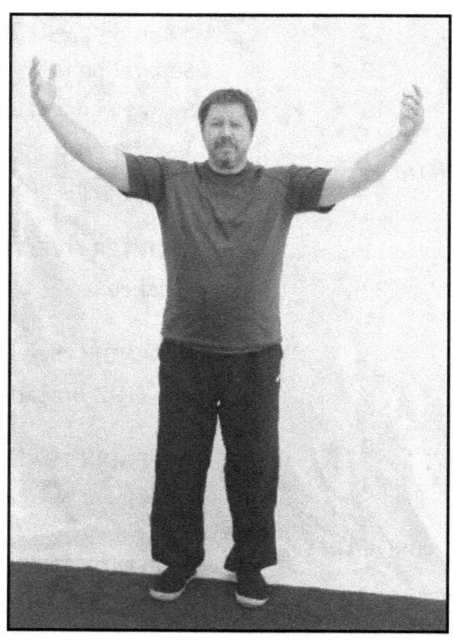

INTRODUCTION

I've always been interested in fitness and movement. As a child I practiced judo, boxing and football. I became less interested in "conventional" sports, so when the Bruce Lee and Kung Fu boom hit in the 70s, it totally captured my interest and imagination. Martial arts, and Chinese Kung Fu (gong fu) in particular, seemed to contain all the different aspects that I was looking for. Physical exercise, combined with fighting, self defence, health, meditation and philosophy.

I began training in Yang Family Tai Chi Chuan (Taijiquan) at the age of 17. I was lucky to find one of the few traditional schools around - at that time genuine gongfu was still something of a rarity in the West, though the boom produced many bandwagon jumpers. I studied Taiji and associated arts in great depth and was lucky to be able to train under many excellent teachers (sifus) and also some "interesting" characters!

One of the best teachers I studied with was Professor Ji Jian Cheng. Sifu Ji Jian-Cheng is Director of Martial Arts and Qigong at Zhejiang University, is graded as 7th Degree level Master of Wushu, is a National Wushu Master for China and a National Referee. He is expert in a number of Chinese martial art systems as well

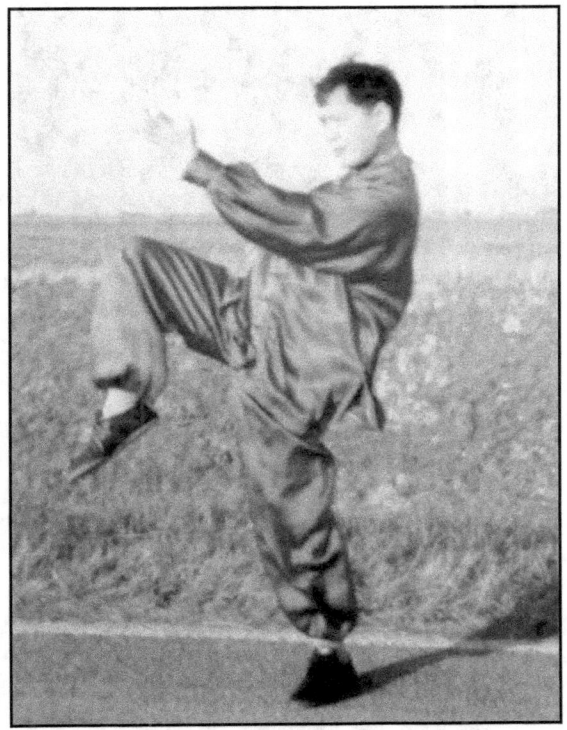

SIFU JI JIAN CHENG

as associated Chi Kung (qigong) practices. Above all, he is an excellent teacher and a very nice man! If you get the chance, I highly recommend training with him.

It was from Sifu Ji that I learned The Eight Brocades and some other methods. The version in this book is largely as Sifu Ji taught, with some minor changes.

Around the year 2000 I became aware of a Russian martial art called Systema. This was something virtually unknown outside of Russia at the time. Even inside Russia it was rare, due

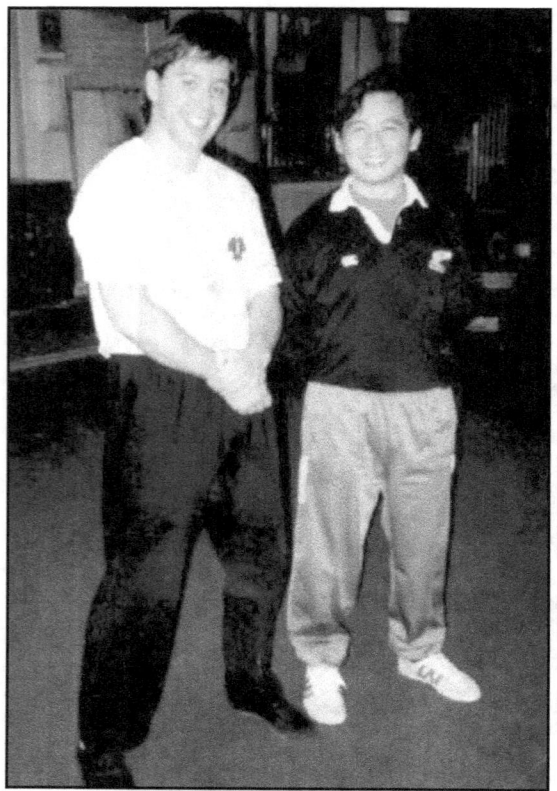

THE AUTHOR WITH SIFU JI JIAN CHENG

partly to its background of use by various specialised military units. I was fortunate enough to meet and train with one of the leading masters, Vladimir Vasiliev, on his first visit to the UK. Vladimir demonstrated such a high level of mastery that I began training in his art, later also visiting Moscow to train with his teacher, Mikhail Ryabko. As might be expected in such an holistic art, Systema also incorporates a wide range of movement, health and breathing practices. I have included some of these here as they dovetail into and complement the Eight Brocades perfectly. They also supply a slightly different viewpoint from the traditional Chinese model, which, for me, gives an interesting contrast.

SIMPLY FLOW

When all is said and done, good movement is good movement and anything that promotes true health is to be applauded. To this end, in 2018 I founded the *Simply Flow Training Program*. This was partly in response to having a lot of friends around the same age (50 something!) asking me about the best way to keep fit and active as they got older. After research into what was available (largely weight training/body sculpting or more extreme types of workout), I set about formulating a "basics up" program that could be practiced by people of any age or experience. The prime factors that I wanted to highlight and promote in the program are what I see as the two fundamental aspects of fitness, both of which become increasingly important as we age: mobility and tension.

Mobility, in brief, is our ability to move and operate as a fully functional human being. Barring injury, disease or disability, there is no real reason why we should not be as mobile at 70 as we were at 7. That may seem like a bold statement but I stand by it. The reason that many people are not so mobile is down to the second aspect, tension. Tension has many causes. Stress, worry and concern, it may be about financial stress, relationships or just from reading the news. It can all have a much bigger impact on our health and fitness than we may imagine.

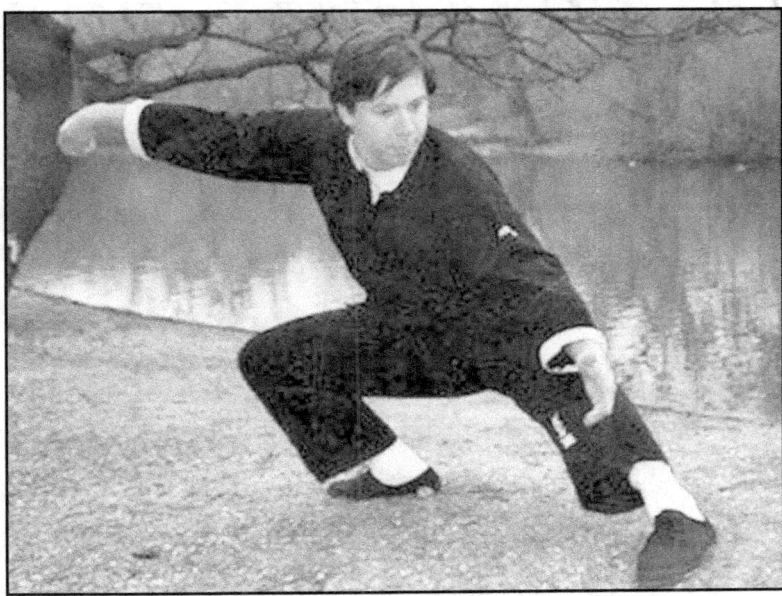

THE AUTHOR PRACTICING TAI CHI CHUAN

Prolonged exposure to even low levels of stress has a serious detrimental effect on our immune system, creates muscular tension throughout the body, affects sleep patterns and can have a negative impact on our work and relationships.

Physical tension can result from poor posture, lifestyle habits, injury, lack of activity, or doing the wrong type of activity. Some fitness methods actively introduce more tension into the body, which can result in problems. Remember the "feel the burn" fitness fads from a while back? Or some of the current big name fitness methods which encourage people to constantly go "fast and hard"? Visually impressive but potentially physically damaging.

The Eight Brocades are one part of the *Simply Flow* syllabus. We teach them in our Tai Chi classes as well as at workshops. They consist of a set of quite straightforward movements which bring benefits on multiple levels. They can be practiced alone or as part of a wider program.

HOW TO USE THIS BOOK

I advise you work through this book movement by movement and get a good feel for the exercises. There is no need to rush any of the movements and this is not a "numbers based" system. By that I mean that the emphasis is on quality rather than quality. You will get more benefit from doing five "proper"

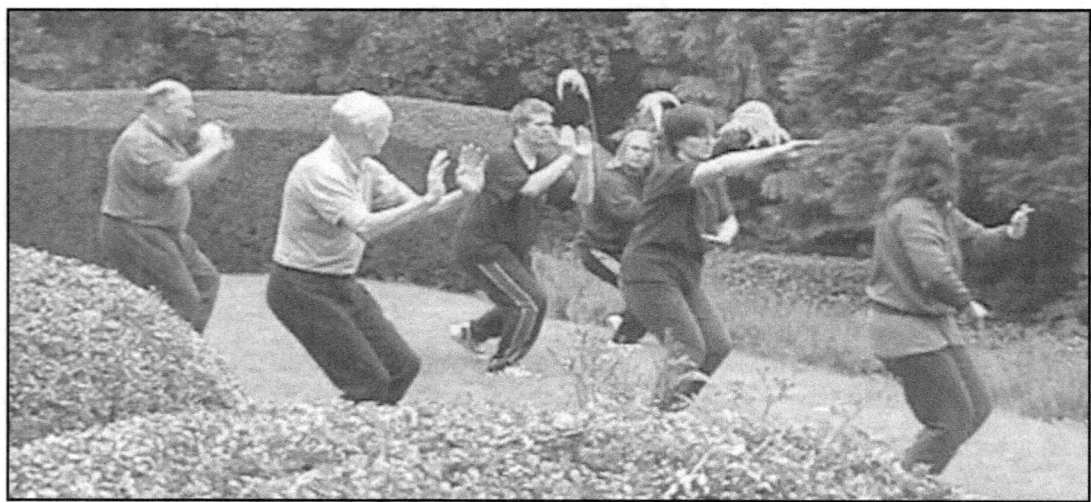

movements than rushing through twenty reps.

If there are any exercises that you feel uncomfortable doing, or that do not suit your current condition, then feel free to give them a miss. If at any time you feel pain or severe discomfort while doing an exercise, then please cease it immediately. If in doubt, always check with your Doctor before trying any new exercise plan. If you have an existing medical condition or injury, then work within its restrictions, do not attempt to "blast through" it. Many of the exercises here can adapted to suit most conditions with a little thought.

A quick note on spelling. Many terms from Chinese medicine and martial arts are used throughout this book. For the most part I have adopted the current standard English spellings, with some of the older variations mentioned too. In short, Tai Chi, Taiji, Taijiquan, etc all refer to the same thing.

QIGONG

The Eight Brocades come under the category of what are called *qigong* (Chi Kung) exercises. Qigong can be literally translated as *Energy Work*. However, Chinese names and titles carry more than one meaning, so let's break the phrase down.

Qi /Chi means "energy". That, in itself, is a rather vague term, but we can think of it in this way; our bodies run on energy. One of the main sources of energy is breathing. From that perspective, qigong is very much concerned with developing good breathing practices.

Energy also comes from food, so diet, herbal medicines and so on form another important aspect of qigong training

Qi is also the term used to describe the body's *intrinsic energy* (see later section on Traditional Chinese Medicine).

Gong means "work." Most people have heard the word from the term gongfu/ Kung Fu, which has come to mean Martial Arts. In fact, Gong Fu actually means "hard work" or "developed skill." A person can have Gong Fu in cooking, or art, or any other discipline or endeavour. The more correct term for Chinese Martial Arts is *Wu Shu* (martial skill).

The ancient Chinese developed a form of writing using pictograms rather than an alphabet. To create these characters in the traditional way can only be achieved with focus, flowing movement and a steady hand. In this sense, traditional brush writing can be practiced as form of qigong in itself.

The symbolic nature of calligraphy means that just even a single character can be loaded with meaning beyond the basic level. If we look at the character for Qi, for example, we find it has two components. Below is the character for cooking rice. Above is the character for steam rising.

This points to one of the main concepts of qigong, which is developing the lower energy centre (*Dantian*) from which qi is circulated up and around the body.

Qigong is quite a modern term, it was coined to cover a wide and varied range of exercises and methods. Qigong practices can range from quiet, static meditation, through to soft, slow and gentle movements coordinated with breathing, through to more intense "hard" conditioning methods, where the body is repeatedly struck with iron bars and similar!

Qigong is practiced for exercise, for religious/ spiritual purposes, as part of martial art training or as treatment for various medical conditions. Generally, all methods are characterised by a focus on harmonising

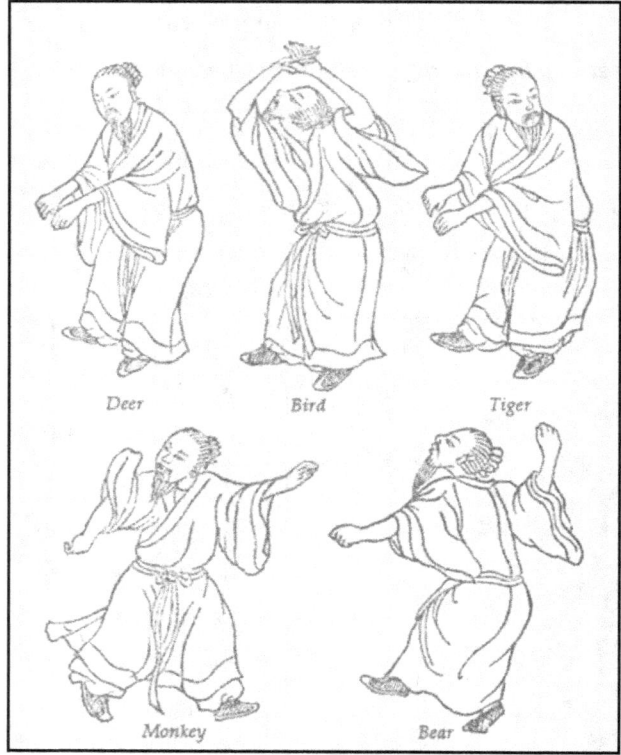

external movements of the body with internal focus, breathing and flow.

The earliest known qigong-like movements were animal dances, performed by ancient Chinese shamans. These have been found depicted in carved art throughout China, going as far back as Neolithic times. From a slightly later time, archaeologists discovered a silk panel with captions as well as picture detailing qigong movements.

The Book of Changes (*I Ching*), written around 1122 B.C., first recorded the concept of qi. Around 450 B.C., Lao Tzu, the founder of Taoism, described breathing techniques in his book *Dao De Jing*. It is from this period that Traditional Chinese Medicine (TCM) began to be developed. Huang Ti's *Yellow Emperor's Classic of Internal Medicine* first appeared in around 300 B.C. and is still considered the bible of Chinese medicine.

From circa 200 B.C. to 500 A.D., Buddhism and yoga meditation techniques were brought from India into China and absorbed into Chinese culture. These techniques, along with native Taoist methods, brought new life to qigong and deepened its practice. However, many teachings were kept secret and were passed down to only a handful of chosen disciples in each generation. For hundreds of years, they were never taught to the layperson.

Circa 500 A.D. a Buddhist monk named Bodhidarma, travelled from India to the Shaolin Temple in China (where he was called Da Mo). He is credited with bringing together the spiritual and martial practices of qigong. He saw how the Shaolin monks had become physically weak through their sedentary meditation practices and so taught them how to strengthen their bodies through movement.

From this developed the famous Shaolin martial arts, internal fighting methods that evolved into powerful self defence systems. These, too, were kept secret and taught only within the temples.

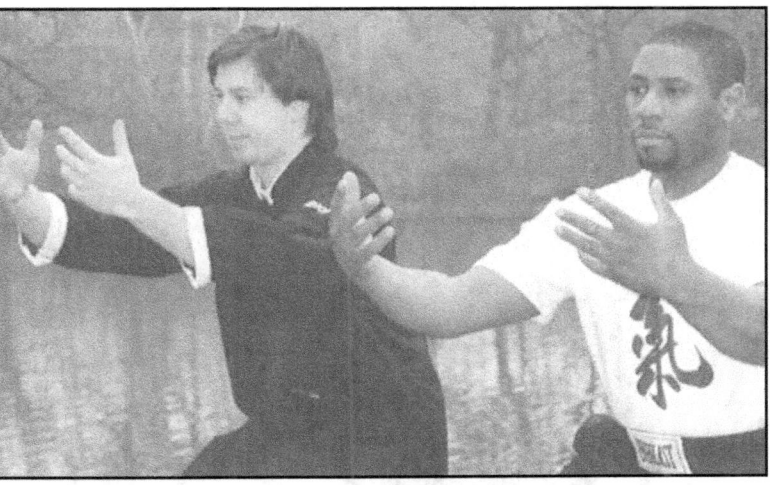

The secrecy around qigong led to thousands of different styles developing. Each family or village, each religious or martial-arts group, developed their own practices separately, suited for their own particular purposes, and passed down only within their own lineage.

For the general population, qigong was just apart of TCM. Many of the famous TCM physicians were also qigong masters. Qigong was their treatment of choice, and if that practice wasn't enough to restore balance, the physician would also prescribe herbs and/or acupuncture.

A huge cultural change occurred in the 20th century following the Cultural Revolution. There was a move to modernise society and ancient practices like TCM were questioned and devalued. Anything remotely connected with religion was politically taboo. Anyone involved in prohibited pursuits would likely be put in jail.

Fortunately, revolutionary leaders fairly soon realized that it was wise to continue TCM and so bans were lifted on qigong. Western influences and technology were also coming more and more into China. Many began to advocate using science and technology to research qigong and TCM.

In 1985, the Chinese government set up the *China Qigong Science Association*. Since then, hundreds of controlled scientific studies of qigong have been carried out, all showing positive benefits of the practice. Qigong was being taught openly at this time, and by 1992 it was estimated that 70-80 million Chinese were practitioners.

During the 1990's qigong began to spread throughout the world. There were international conferences in Berkeley, California (1990) and in Vancouver, Canada

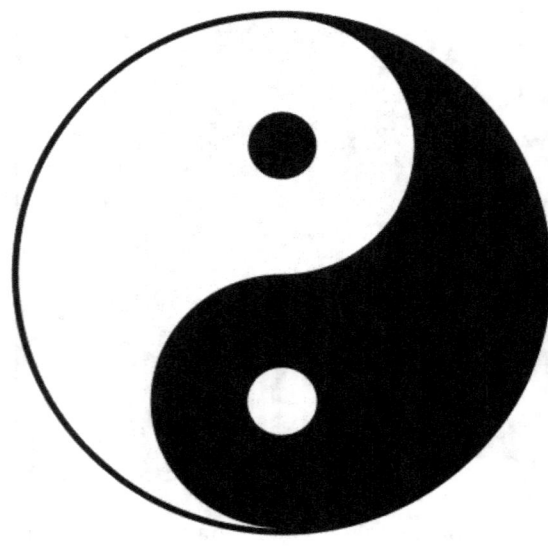

(1995). By 1996, there were more than one thousand published articles available in English on different aspects of qigong research.

In 1997, it was estimated that there were over 100,000 qigong practitioners outside of China. The practice has continued to grow since, making qigong, alongside yoga, one of the most popular forms of health exercise in the world today.

All Chinese martial arts have their own qigong methods, or can be practiced as qigong (such as Taijiquan). A few examples of distinct stand-alone styles are: Six Healing Sounds, Five Animal Frolics, Five Elements, Eight Pieces of Brocade, Swimming Dragon, and Daoyin.

TRADITIONAL CHINESE MEDICINE

TCM is a system of medical care that developed in China over thousands of years. It takes quite a different approach to Western medicine, seeking to treat a person as a whole and looking at being preventative as well as curative. TCM uses a combination of practices including:

- herbal remedies
- acupuncture and acupressure
- moxibustion (burning herbs)
- massage therapy
- feng shui
- qigong
- cupping
- diet

TCM is based on a number of concepts, all of which are deeply rooted in Chinese culture and philosophy.

YIN YANG

Yin and yang is an ancient concept which can be traced back to the Shang dynasty (1600–1100 BC). Yin and yang represent the two complementary aspects that every phenomenon in the universe can be divided into. It is said that the idea first took root by someone watching the sunny and shady side of a hill and how the two changed.

The yin-yang symbol is a circle divided into two parts. The white part is yang, the dark part is yin. So the sun-facing hill side would be yang and the shady side yin. Other attributions include:

YIN	YANG
Night	Day
Female	Male
Cold	Hot
Moon	Sun

Yin and yang are interdependent; you need yin to have yang, and yang to have yin. Think about running and rest, for example. After running for a while we get tired and need to rest, so that we have energy to start running again. Yang activity is dependent on the yin activity yin is dependent on yang: if we aren't already moving, we can't stop and rest. In this way, yin-yang is always in balance.

As we see from the symbol, as one side reaches its fullest point, it is already starting to diminish. Think of the sun at noon, at its highest point in the sky is when it begins its descent. The balance is maintained by the constant interaction and flow between the two states. If that relationship goes out of balance, then problems arise!

Looking at the diagram we also see that yin contains a seed of yang (in the form of a white dot) and vice-versa. This is part of the balance, pointing to the fact that everything contains some aspect of its opposite. In a relationship of harmony, the two energies

 ## Disease Development from Yin Yang Perspective

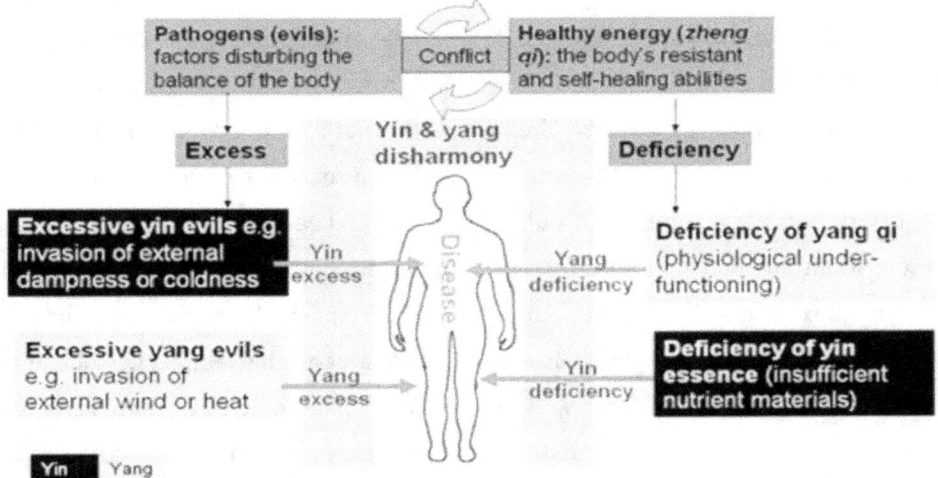

CLASSIFICATION OF THINGS ACCORDING TO THE THEORY OF THE FIVE ELEMENTS

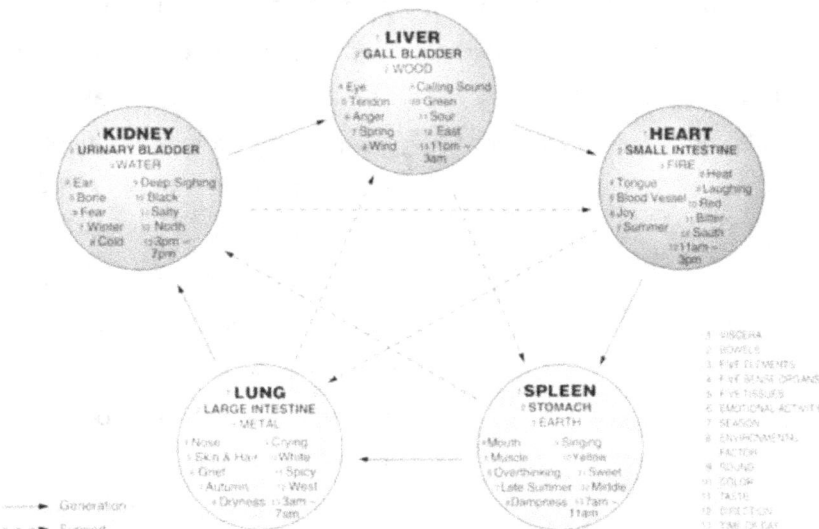

blend into one seamless whole, representing the dynamic flow of the natural world.

The concept of yin and yang is also applied to the human body; for example, the upper body is yang, while the lower body is yin in character.

Yin and yang is also applied to body functions, as well as disease symptoms. Cold and heat sensations are viewed as yin and yang symptoms, respectively. So yang/ heat sensations might include night sweats, insomnia, dry throat, dark urine, rapid pulse. Yin/ cold sensations might include shivers, cold limbs, pale complexion, diarrhoea, weak pulse. They might also be applied to emotional issues, such as anger, feeling listless and so on. A TCM physician seeks to restore the body's natural flow and balances by using the various treatment methods.

FIVE ELEMENT THEORY

Chinese philosophy also classifies things using the Five Element model. The Five Elements are a template that organises all natural phenomena into five groups or patterns. Each of the five groups - Wood, Fire, Earth, Metal, and Water - includes categories such as a season, a direction, climate, stage of growth and development, internal organ, body tissue, emotion, taste, colour, sound and so on.

Everything within each element is related. Take Water as an example. Looking at the Five Element diagram, we see that Water is related to winter, cold climate, the north, the colour black, the Kidneys. We also see in the diagram a cycle of creation and a cycle of destruction. In basic terms, wood is consumed by fire, which create earth. Water nourishes wood but destroys fire.

This basic idea is extended into the function of bodily organs. TCM, uses the Five Element principle to help maintain the balance between the organs, obviously the process of each has a direct effect on the next organ in the chain.

MERIDIANS

We have already spoken a little about the concept of qi / chi. TCM sees this as the vital life force that inhabits the body of every living thing. This is divided into pre-natal qi (the amount of energy that we are born with) and post-natal qi (the energy we get from food, breathing and our environment.) Qi is in a constant state of flow around the body. Think of it is as electrical energy that powers the body's functions and systems.

According to TCM, qi travels around the body in meridians. These pathways were mapped by physicians and martial artists over the years, and it was found that manipulating certain points on a meridian could have an effect on the body. So massaging a point may bring relief from pain, for example. On the

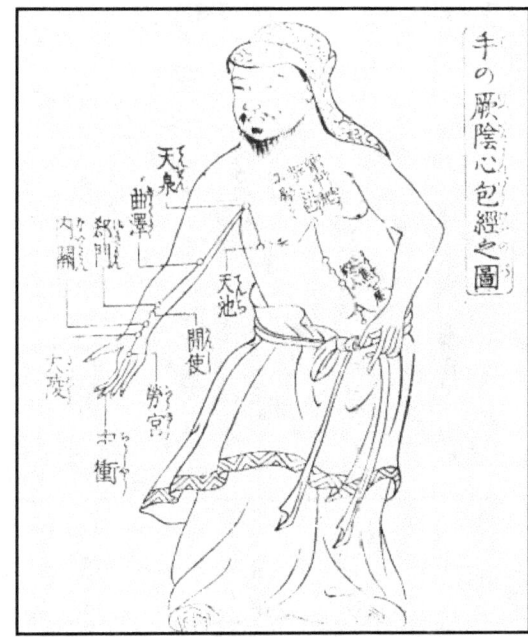

other hand, striking a point in a certain way might result in a knock out or a "draining of energy".

The meridian system is most widely used in acupuncture, where slim needles are inserted into specific points along a meridian in order to strengthen the flow of energy. That flow may also be strengthened by specific qigong exercises, where the mind and breath are used to direct qi into various parts of the body. Some also claim that qi can be extended beyond the body, passed from one person to another in order to facilitate healing.

These, then, are the primary theories underpinning TCM, albeit explained very

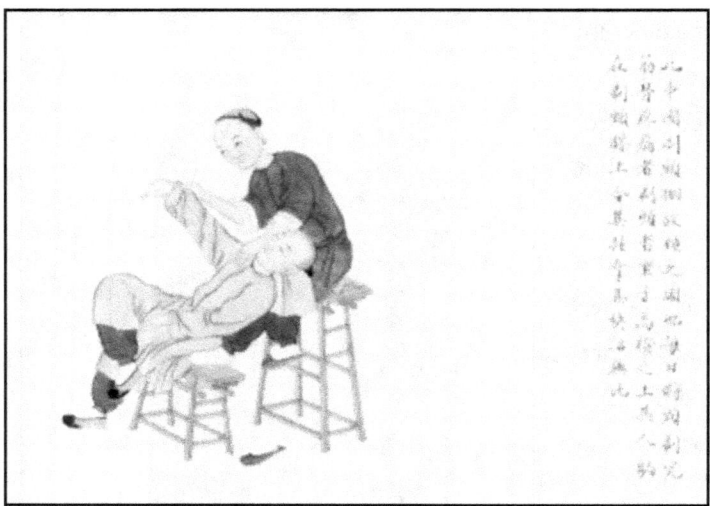

briefly and at a basic level! I would encourage you, if interested, to research further, there are numerous good books on the subject.

How much of this theory is accepted by Western science is another issue. There are certainly aspects of TCM that are questionable (use of tiger bones, for example). However, Western science is also now beginning to understand and explore the complex and profound relationship between mind and body. There have been numerous studies on the positive effects of good breathing, the benefits of exercises such as Taiji in helping the healing process and so on. Acupuncture is widely spread now, often prescribed as a complement to Western medicine.

My own view is that it is not necessary to fully understand or even believe in any of the theories, as presented. I describe them here mostly in order to give some background to the exercises that follow. The important thing, for me, is what you gain from the the exercises. Do they make you feel better? Do you find your mobility improving, do you feel more energetic and "alive" after practice? That is the first stage. Then, if you wish, you can research the various different theories and explanations as to what may be happening!

For example, some discount the meridian theory but talk of an "energy field" surrounding the body, which can be strengthened by exercise, diet and so on.

Similarly, we have mentioned the connection of some of the qigong methods to religious / spiritual practices (usually Buddhist or Taoist). Spiritual belief, of any type, is very much a personal issue and I would like to make it clear that there is no belief system associated in this presentation of the Eight Brocade methods, nor is any necessary to get the physical benefits of the exercises. They are

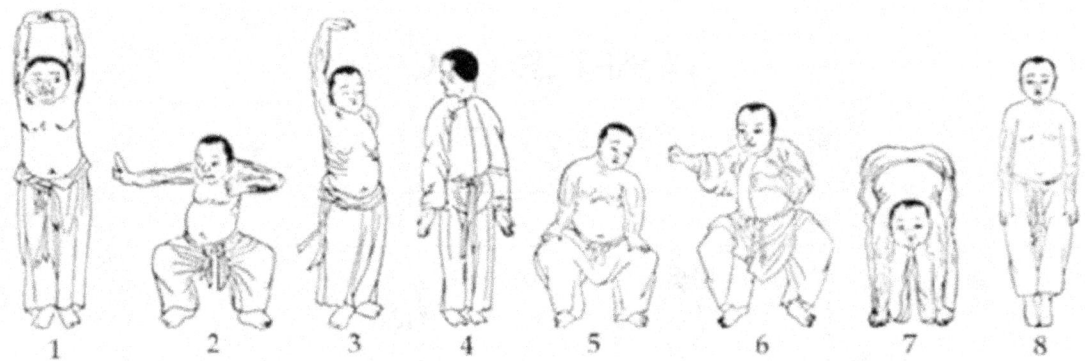

taught here purely an exercise system with no religious connotations.

THE EIGHT BROCADES

The Eight Brocade Exercise (*Baduanjin*) has its roots in ancient qigong practices. The name refers to eight movements, each of which is seen as a "treasure". A brocade in ancient China was an intricately woven piece of silk, an item of great value. So another term for the exercise might be The Eight Treasures. However the mention of silk also gives us an important idea about how the exercises are performed.

Silk is soft but very strong. In many cultures it was worn under armour in order to resist blades. So silk is not only decorative it is functional. Not only sleek and soft, but strong. This informs us as to how the Eight Brocades should be practiced - smoothly but with intention and focus.

The exercise was first mentioned in the Song Dynasty c. 1150. The *Ten Compilations on Cultivating Perfection* (c. 1300) features illustrations of all eight movements. Nineteenth century sources attribute the exercises to legendary folk hero General Yue Fei. The legend claims he taught the exercise to his troops to help keep them strong and prepared for battle.

Whatever the origins, the Eight Brocades have come down to us through the generations and are one of the more widely practiced qigong sets. This does mean that there are variations in the movements, so what you see here may be slightly different from other versions. That is generally true of most Chinese disciplines, however, as over the years, successive masters add their own touch or "signature moves" to an exercise. The most important thing is that the underlying principles are adhered to, so it is those that we shall examine next.

CHAPTER TWO
FUNDAMENTALS

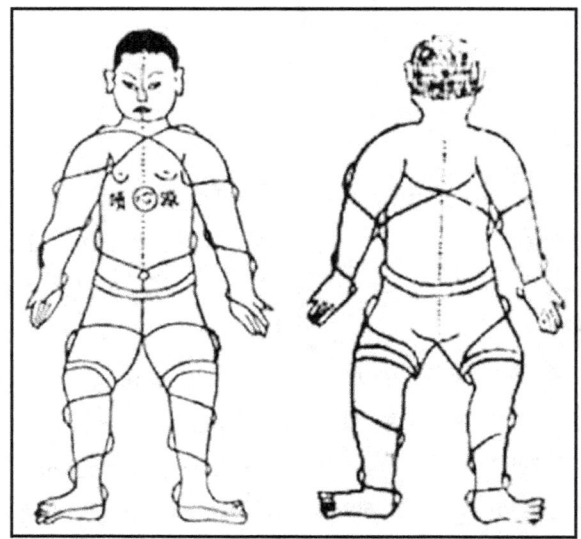

FUNDAMENTALS

The principles of good movement vary little across any exercise or movement discipline. There are many treatises in Chinese martial arts, such as Yang Cheng Fu's *Ten Essentials of Tai Chi Chuan*, which go into great detail on all aspects of movement. However, in terms of brevity and accessibility, I prefer to use the model from the Russian art of Systema - the Four Pillars. These are easy to understand (though not always to do perfectly!) and can be applied to any type of exercise. Or any type of movement, come to that, for we should be aware of these principles throughout our daily activities.

THE FOUR PILLARS

The Four Pillars are breathing, movement, relaxation and posture. I think of each of these as the four legs of a chair; each must be present and of the right length, otherwise we wobble! The four are, of course, closely inter-related, but to keep things clear, let's first examine each in turn to help you understand its role.

BREATHING

The most fundamental Pillar, for without breath there is no life! We can go without food and water days or weeks, but most people struggle to hold their breath for even a couple of minutes. Breathing is a largely unconscious activity which goes on 24/7 and that is where the problems begin. We lose touch with our breathing and, consequently, it becomes less effective and efficient as we age. Again, medical conditions aside, there is no need for this to happen. Re-establishing conscious contact with our breathing is the first step to improved health and fitness.

The breath also acts as a very strong two-way bridge between our internal/emotional state and our external/physical state. When used correctly, the breath connects the two and allows one to influence the other. This makes breath work our primary method of stress management and fear control. Breathing can also be used to power movement and bring an element of mindfulness to our exercises. This mindfulness opens the door to the meditative aspects of our practice and, even at a basic level, is a powerful antidote to daily worries and stress.

Unless otherwise directed, the standard breathing procedure is to inhale through the nose and exhale through the mouth. Breathing should be comfortable, not over filling the lungs or completely emptying them, unless otherwise directed. Learn to breathe smoothly and to the requirements of the situation. When you first start out, it is advisable to practice breathing in a safe and comfortable position. If you have any blood pressure or other health issues, always

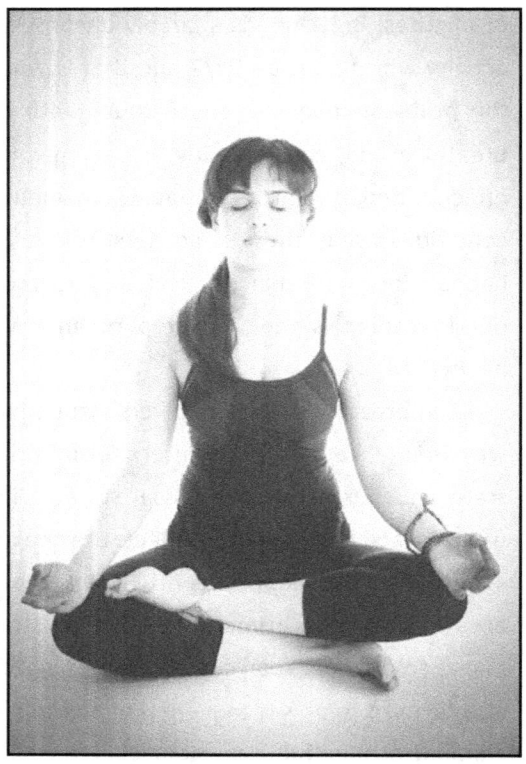

be sure check with your doctor prior to training.

There are three basic depths of breathing. The first is shallow or burst breathing. Think of a dog panting, the breath comes in the nose and straight out of the mouth. This is most often used as a recovery breath, or in stressful situations. If your system is stressed you can use burst breathing to regain control and return to a state of equilibrium.

The second is our everyday chest breathing. The ribcage expands and contracts with each inhale and exhale. This may still be fairly shallow, or can be practiced more deeply. The main point to watch is that there is no unnecessary tension on the inhale, particularly in the shoulders.

The third is abdominal breathing. This is where the diaphragm is fully used in order to draw and expel the breath. This can be "normal", where the diaphragm pushes out on the inhale, in on the exhale, or "reverse breathing" where the diaphragm pulls in and up on the inhale and expands out on the exhale.

We recommend you begin with chest breathing, with burst breathing for recovery. Deeper breathing will come with time as your body relaxes. Never force the breath and if at any time you feel dizzy, then come out of the exercise immediately and sit quietly to recover.

We use shapes to describe our breathing exercise and the first pattern we look at is Circular Breathing. One half of the circle is an inhale, the other half an exhale. Each should be equal in length and depth.

The initial aim of CB is to put us back in touch with our breathing. Sit or lay down in a comfortable position. Relax the muscles, particularly around the shoulders. Now, in your own time, inhale to about 80% of your full capacity, then exhale the same way. Don't worry about the length of breathing and be sure not to over-expand or tense the chest.

Take around a dozen breaths in this position, keep it natural, keep it unforced.

You should find that even after a short exercise such as this you will feel more relaxed, both physically and emotionally. This, then, is an ideal exercise for those times during the day when we begin to feel stressed out. Find yourself a quiet place and run through CB for a couple of minutes. This is also good preparation for situations such as going into an interview, having to speak in public, and so on. A minute or so of CB beforehand will help steady the nerves.

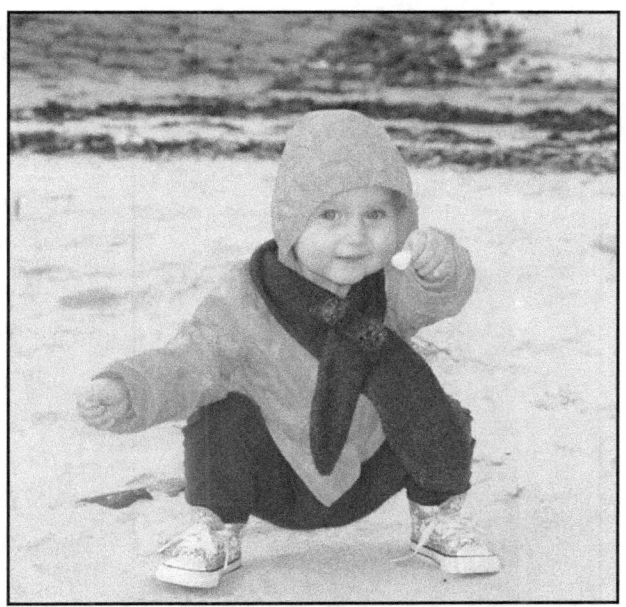

POSTURE

Watch how a toddler sits, watch how they squat or move up and down from the floor. You will notice they have a perfectly straight back and very open hips. As we grow older, posture often deteriorates. This can be due to injury and illness but is more often down to lifestyle, tension and general bad habits.

Improved posture means that we move better, breathe better and place less stress on our joints. It can also help with back issues, which currently account for the loss of millions of working days in the UK.

Good posture simply means keeping the body in balance. It is not about "standing to attention" in a tense, military fashion, but maintaining a relaxed, neutral position - shoulders and hips level, spine straight.

You can check your posture in a mirror. Stand normally and check to see if your shoulders tilt, if your hips are level. When you sit, try and keep the back upright and don't let the head sag forward or back as this can cause tension in the neck.

It is very good to get into the habit of monitoring your posture regularly throughout the day. If you are sitting at a desk for a long period of time, every now and then check that you are not hunching, leaning, or tilting the neck, for example.

Here's a simple exercise to check and correct your standing posture.

Stand with feet shoulder width. Check that your feet are parallel and the knees are pointing

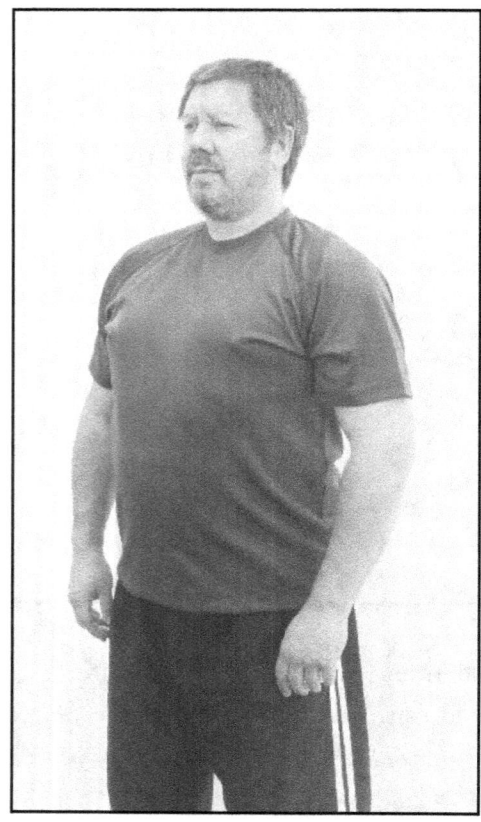

imagine there is a string coming out the crown of your head and you are being suspended from it. Tuck the chin in slightly. Slowly lift the hands above the head, this should help you feel if the body is straight or not.

Now this may sound like a lot of instructions to carry out just to get good posture! But don't worry! The more you do this kind of exercise, the more you will find the body settling into position naturally, without thought. It is exactly the same as our breathing. Bringing back conscious control of our posture allows us to gently correct it and so educate the body as to how it should feel. Checking yourself regularly throughout the day will help a lot too!

forwards. Bring a little tension into the thighs. Now take your hips slightly back - in other words your weight should be sat back a little in your heels, to make sure you are not leaning forward. Relax the upper body but do not slouch.

Allow the shoulders to move back slightly. Imagine you are opening the chest a little. There should be no tension, you should not be in "parade ground" posture, just ensure the spine is straight. Turning the palms forward will give you the right feeling. Now, move the head back a little, to ensure it is not tilted forward. Try to

POOR NECK POSTURE

TILTED BACK

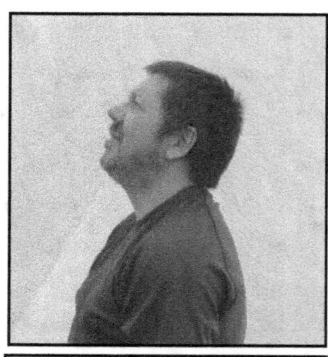

TILTED FORWARD

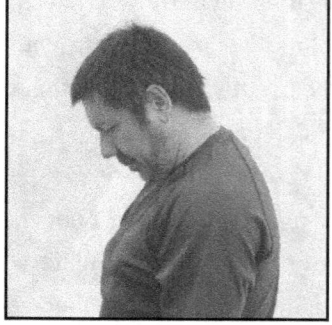

Another great exercise for checking posture and strengthening the legs is the Assisted Squat. This can involve more pressure on the legs so please take things easy at first.

Find a secure, flat surface, such as a wall or a closed door. Stand with your back to it. Bring the feet away from the wall a little and to a comfortable position, usually just over shoulder width apart. The toes must point in the same direction as the knees. They may be pointing straight forward, or be turned out a little, though not pointing inwards.

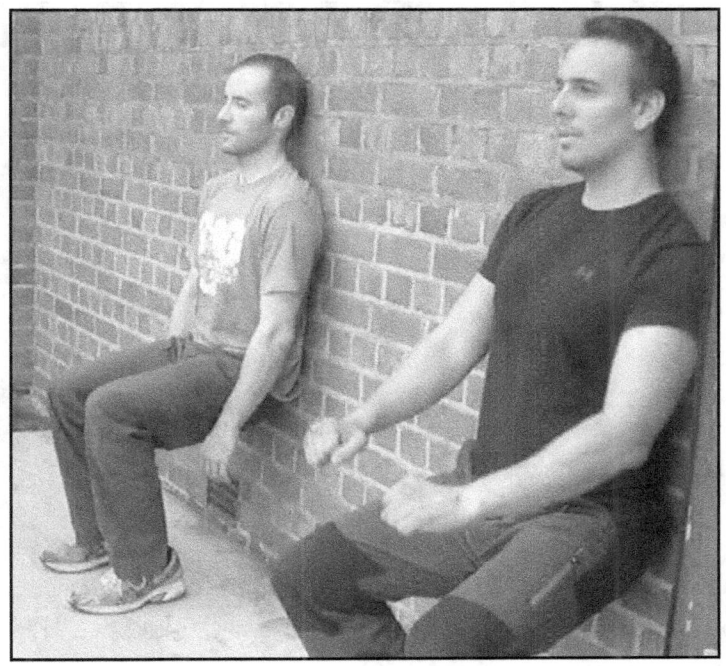

Inhale, then on an exhale, slowly bend the knees and lower yourself down. Just go to your comfortable range of motion at first. The trick is to maintain the alignment of the body, so the back should remain in full contact with the supporting surface, from shoulders to tailbone. If you tuck the tailbone in a little and tilt the pelvis slightly, you will find it more comfortable. Hold for a second as you inhale, then exhale and straighten up again.

Repeat this a few times. As your strength builds and the hips open, you will be able to sink lower into the squat. You can also try going down and holding the position for a few minutes - a great one for the thigh muscles!

RELAXATION

"Relax" is a very loaded word . It usually conjures up images of sitting on the couch with a beer, not something that most exercise coaches condone! *Simply Flow* uses the term relax more as a measure of how much tension there is in the body. Basically, we are always looking to operate with the minimal amount of tension necessary to complete the task.

Why? Because unwanted tension creates restriction and damage! Think of tension as salt. We need salt to survive, so we add a pinch here and there to our food. But too much salt creates problems, raises blood pressure and so on. Similarly, who would pour half a pot of salt onto their ice cream? We use it as and when

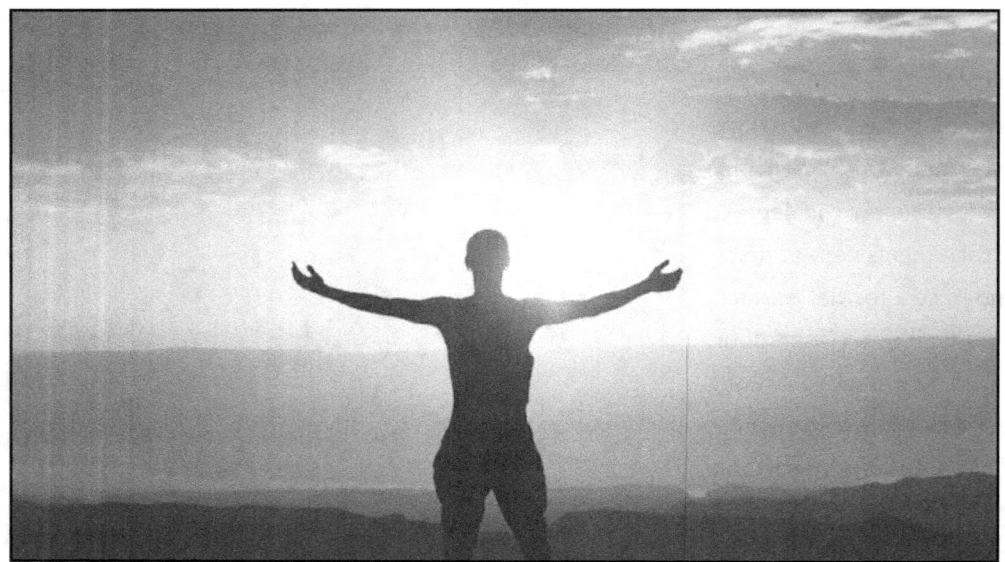

necessary (although, of course, modern processed foods often contain much more salt and sugar than we are aware of.)

The same principle applies with tension. If the body is completely relaxed, it cannot move and we are laying on the floor. Even to stand takes a measure of tension. Yet how many people stand with buttocks clenched, hips tight, with a slight lean, shoulder raised, forehead creased in worry? And all you are doing is standing! This kind of tension restricts breathing and blood flow and inhibits movement. When fast movement is carried out under tension, we run the risk of injury (as in the more dangerous forms of exercise).

Tension is closely related to posture and fixing one will usually fix the other. So again, get into the habit of monitoring tension levels throughout the day. That also includes your emotional tension - negative thoughts and stress contribute greatly to physical tension!

Learning to release tension and relax into our movement gives us efficiency and and flow. Watch how cats move in everyday activity, smooth and fluid.

Here's a great exercise that uses our breathing to work on tension/relaxation. We will work our Circular Breathing again and the procedure is to tense on the inhale, relax on the exhale. We also use Selective Tension for this exercise, which means that we only tense a particular muscle group, the rest of the body stays relaxed. You can work round all the major muscle groups of the body, but for now, we will just work the shoulders.

Find a comfortable position, standing, sitting or prone. Inhale nose, exhale mouth for a while, slowing the breathing. Then, on the inhale, bunch up and tense the shoulders. Just the shoulders, remember! On the exhale, completely relax the shoulders, just let them drop. Repeat a few times. We are conditioning the body to release tension every time we exhale, the tension goes away with the breath! Again, this is a great exercise to do as soon as you feel unwanted tension creeping into the shoulders, especially if you are sitting at a computer all day.

MOVEMENT

Bio-mechanically, we are little different from the animals we share the world with, particularly mammals and apes. We take in information through our senses and interact with our environment through movement. Even speech is a function of breathing and movement. As children we run, fall, climb, swim, jump and roll. There are very few inhibitions on our movement. As we grow older, those inhibitions grow. It may be that we drive to work, spend all day sitting at a desk, drive home again and sit on the couch all night. It may be that tension "freezes" our shoulders and they become more and more hunched.

In short, use it or lose it! As I said before, medical reasons aside, there is no reason to have lesser mobility as we grow older. There are numerous studies that show how maintaining mobility reduces the effects of

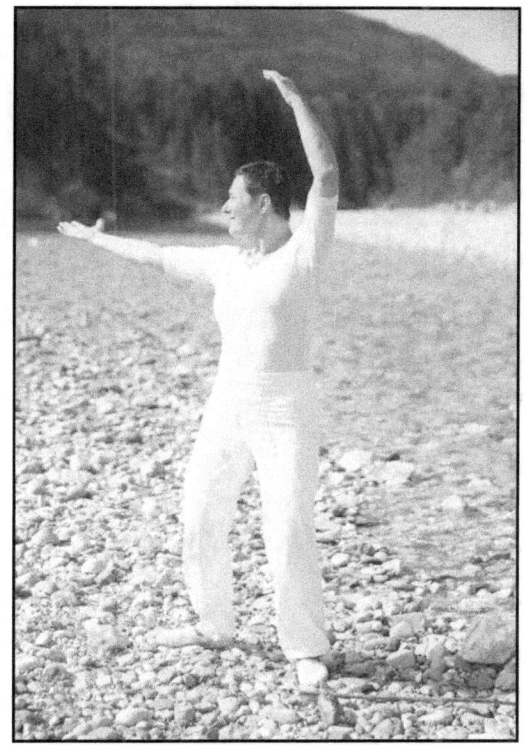

ageing. That includes good range of motion, flexibility, smoothness of movement, and so on.

Mobility is the ability to move ourselves in an efficient and effective way; a way that minimises impact and wear on the body but allows us to complete our task successfully, whatever it may be. Under the *Simply Flow* approach, there is no distinction in what you use your movement for. Be it exercise, sports, dancing, martial arts, swimming or just everyday activities, it is all the same process. Our exercise should be natural and free, so that our training truly prepares us for life!

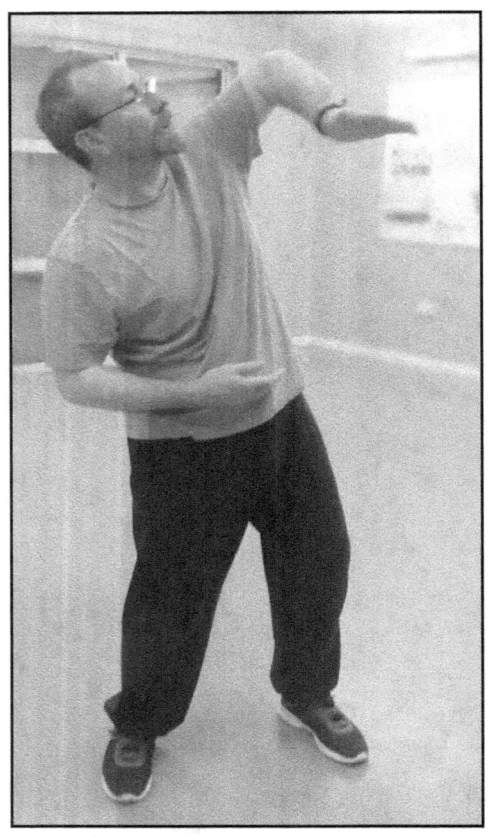

A simple preparation for movement is to practice some joint rotation exercises. Work through all the joints of the body in turn and moving them in gentle circles. I usually start with the head and work down. If you have no neck issues, let the chin drop, then slowly rotate the head in each direction. Next, circle the shoulders, the elbows, the wrists. From here, work down into the hips. Finally, seated or standing on one leg, rotate ankle, knee and hip. Remember to work slowly and to your comfortable range of motion.

INTEGRATION

When you practice the Eight Brocades, bear the Four Pillars in mind. While we have just separated them out, you should always be aware that they are holistic and interdependent. You can't breathe well with poor posture and poor breathing will bring tension into the body. Work each Pillar step by step.

There is what we could call a Fifth Pillar, which is the combination of all the other four working smoothly and efficiently together. Sports people often call this "being in the zone", some call it mindfulness, others the "flow state." Martial artists experience it as being "in the moment" and acting instinctually and powerfully in a dangerous situation.

If you practice correctly and with diligence, I don't doubt that you will enter this state at certain times, particularly if you are under some kind of pressure, or even just involved in joyful movement. I use the word "joy" deliberately, though it is not something you often hear in the world of exercise, where everything is supposed to be "sweat, struggle and strain."

Our view is that life has enough of those already, why spend your free time chasing them? Think back again to how children behave; they explore and interact, everything is new and exciting. They play, without any thought as to how they look and without any motive other than to enjoy themselves.

Apply the same feeling to your exercise. Learn to move and function with joy, it will have a profound effect on your life as a whole. Now, let's look at some principles specific to the Eight Brocades

STANCE

In traditional Chinese martial arts, the first thing a student does is stand in a stance - often for long periods at a time! The aim was to not only build a strong foundation in the legs, but also to get the student to understand how the upper body should relax down into its base of support. The Eight Brocades uses only three stances, fewer than most of the martial arts but it is nonetheless important to understand what they are and how they work. The stances are all static, ie there is no footwork involved, which makes things a little more straightforward!

UPRIGHT STANCE

The feet are shoulder width apart, toes pointing forward. The knees are straight but not locked. This is what you might call an "everyday" position. It is (or should be!) how you stand naturally. The width of the feet can vary a little to make the position comfortable. For example, in the last of the eight exercises (Bouncing) I prefer to have the feet almost touching.

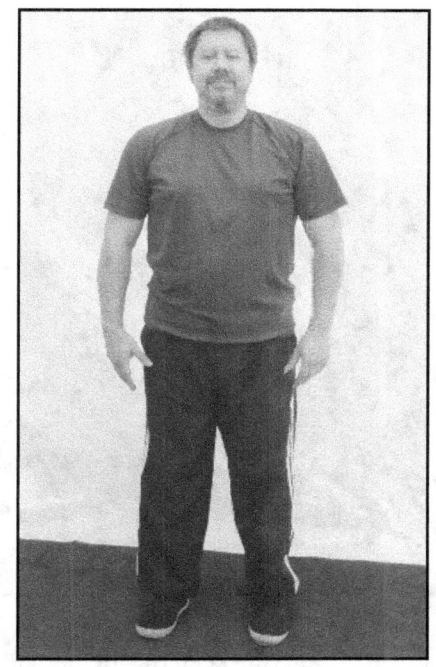

HORSE STANCE

This is a very common stance in Chinese martial arts and is seen as the basis for all others. It is called Horse Stance as it approximates the position of riding a horse. For normal Horse, the feet come out a little wider than shoulder width, the knees are bent and you sit into the posture. For now, the hands can stay on the hips, or if you are feeling "martial" you can hold the fists at the waist.

The most important thing in stance work is to check your alignments. Incorrect alignment, particularly for the knees, can cause problems, so be sure to run through this list, from the feet up.

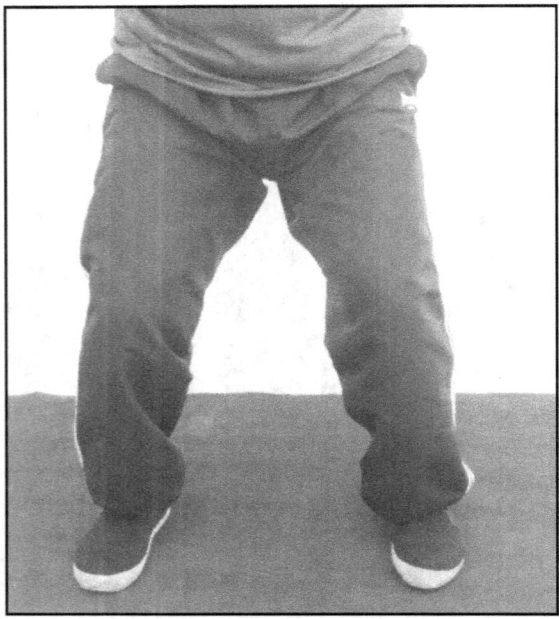

Feet parallel - if you can, keep the feet parallel. Imagine the middle toe on each foot pointing directly forwards. If you find this difficult at first, it is okay to let the toes point out a little but not too far!

Knees in line - it is vital that the knees should point over the toes. The should never point inwards - that will transfer load into the knees rather than through them! Don't sink too low into the posture at first and should you get any sharp knee pain, come out of the posture immediately.

Hips - the hips should be tilted slightly. Tuck the tailbone in a little. Think of the pelvis as a bowl on which the upper body rests.

Spine - the back should be upright, as in our earlier assisted squat exercise. Indeed, that exercises is great preparation for Horse.

Chest - naturally open, not sunken or expanded outwards.

Shoulders - also level and in line with the hips. Make sure they are not tense/lifted or slouched.

Head - the neck is straight, head upright with chin tucked in slightly.

ZHAN ZHUANG

If you wish, you can practice standing in this stance for a short time each day. This is known as *Zhan Zhuang*, or Standing Like a Post. There are variations on foot and hand position but for the basic version work into your stance as above, then raise the hands up to chest height. Keep the shoulders relaxed and the arms rounded, as though you are holding a large ball or jug

Once you are settled in place, work into your Circular Breathing and focus on the inhale/exhale. Allow the breathing to slow and, while maintaining structure, try to let the body relax down into the legs.

Stand like this for a few minutes, then, maintaining the rounded shape, lower the hands to waist height. After the same amount of time, finish by letting the hands drop and

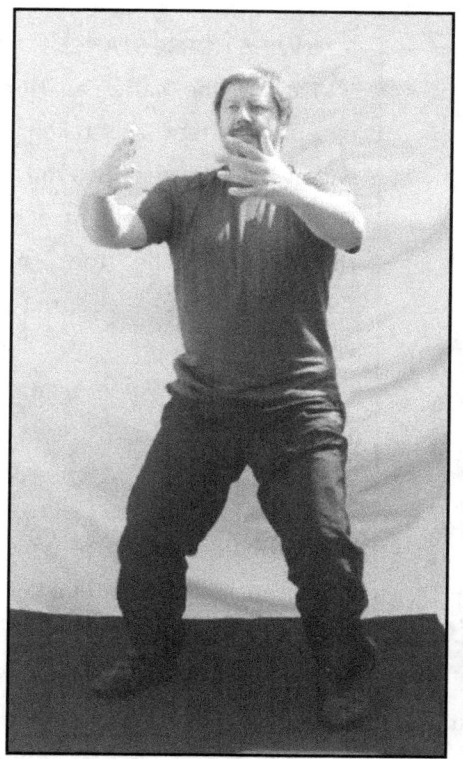 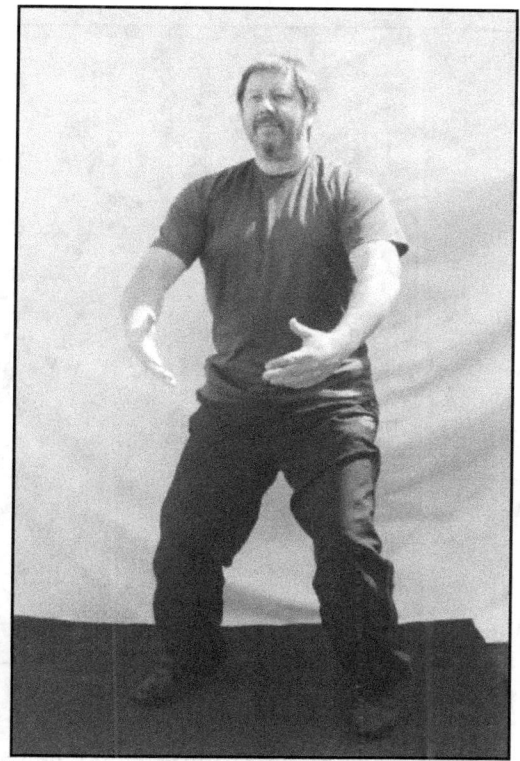

slowly straightening the knees.

Be aware that this posture is far more challenging than it looks, both physically and mentally! On a physical level you will first notice any tension in the body - usually in shoulders, lower back and thighs.

Try and dissolve this tension, let it slip away. Another method of dealing with the tension is to increase it on the inhale (tense the muscle even more) then relax it on the exhale. The tension drains away with the breath. You can adjust the amount of pressure put into the legs by changing the height of the stance, but always check your knee alignment.

On a mental level, you will find all sorts of thoughts flying through your brain. This is perfectly natural, just let them come and go. Do not try and "think of nothing", this is impossible to start! Let the mind naturally settle by focusing on your breathing.

Think of this process as having a jar with some dirt in the bottom. You fill the jar with water, put the lid on and shake it up. The water is now muddy. Put the jar down and eventually the dirt will settle to the bottom and the water become clear again. So, stillness brings clarity.

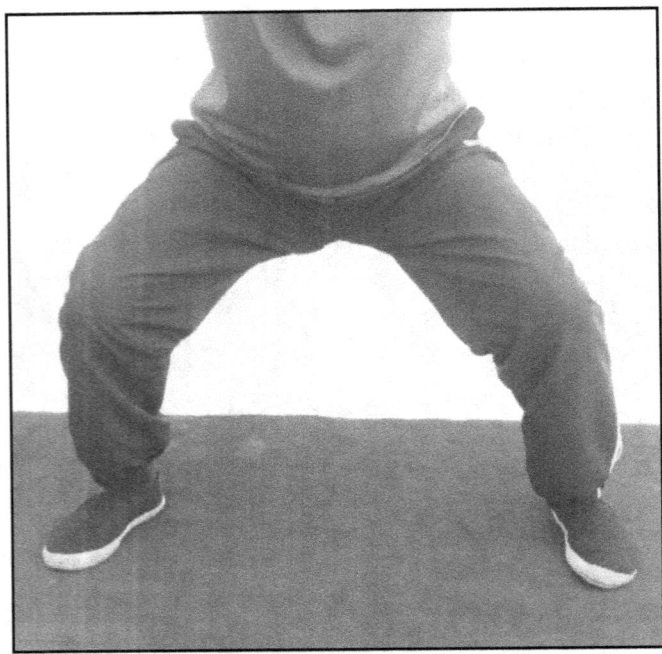

WIDE HORSE STANCE

Exactly the same as Horse, except the feet are taken out wider. In this position you can work to get the thighs parallel to the ground. The toes point forward, or it is okay to turn them slightly outward at first. Remember your knee alignment again!

SPEED

Qigong exercises are typically practiced slowly. If you have ever seen people doing Tai Chi forms you will get the idea. There are a couple of reasons for this. The first is that as you are doing the movements you should be checking through all the postural requirements. As you will have seen, there are a lot of things to pay attention to! If the movements are rushed you may be missing out important details or introducing unnecessary tension into the movements.

The second reason is that all movements should be coordinated with the breathing. This is where the mindful aspect of the exercises comes into play. Now it may be that, at first, you are too busy thinking about the movement to focus on the breathing. That is okay. Get the movement pattern fixed first, then bring in the breathing aspect.

Each movement has a specific inhale/exhale timing, using the Circular Breathing. What you should aim to do is fit the speed of the movement to the length of the breath. Let's try a simple exercise to give you an example.

Pick a simple movement- for example, we will lift the hands from the waist to shoulder height and back down again (this is actually the opening move of the Tai Chi form!) Don't worry about stance, you can do this sitting down.

Start with the hands at waist height as shown. Slowly lift the arms to shoulder height, letting

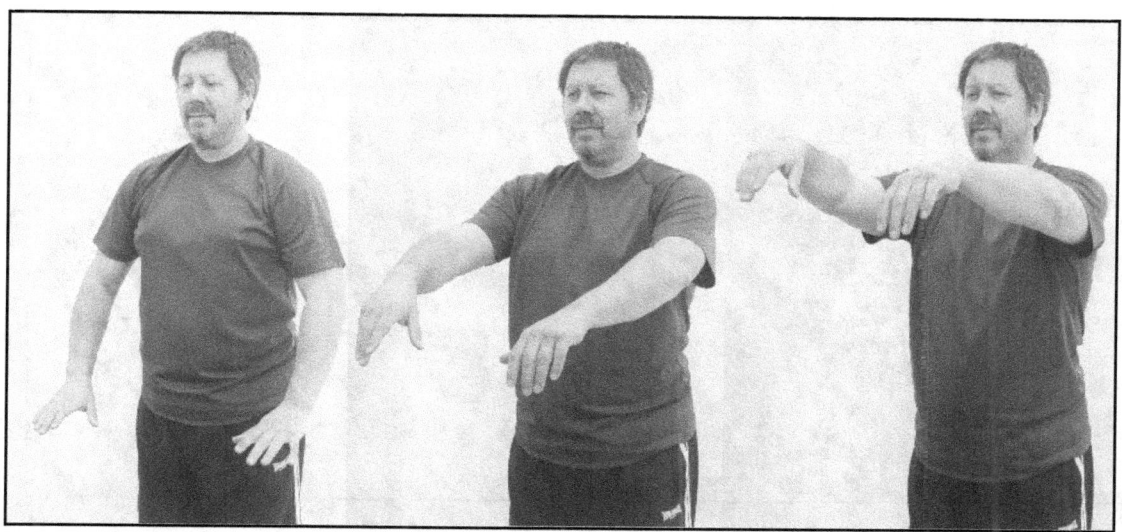

the wrists and fingers relax. Then bring the hands back down to the start position. Run through this a few times.

Now, work into your Circular Breathing. Inhale on the rise and exhale on the fall. Allow the breath to start just before the movement. This way the breathing will lead the movement rather than follow it.

Next, begin to slow the breathing. The hands should move correspondingly slower. Try going as slow as you can and really work to feel that connection between breath and movement. If it helps, you can count as you breathe - for example, in your mind count slowly 1, 2, 3, 4 on each inhale / exhale. This will also help keep your breathing tempo even. Over time you can work up to longer and deeper breaths, this is a method we call Ladder Breathing.

OPEN AND CLOSE

Something very characteristic of Chinese arts is the concept of "movement within movement." One aspect of this is what is called Open and Close. It simply means that during different parts of the movement, certain sections of the body can be expanded or contracted /opened or closed. This adds in extra layers of detail within the movement and leads the way to deeper internal work.

To start to understand this, think of the various parts of the body that can be "open and closed." The most obvious is the chest - after all, the ribcage naturally expands and contracts with every breath, or at least it should!

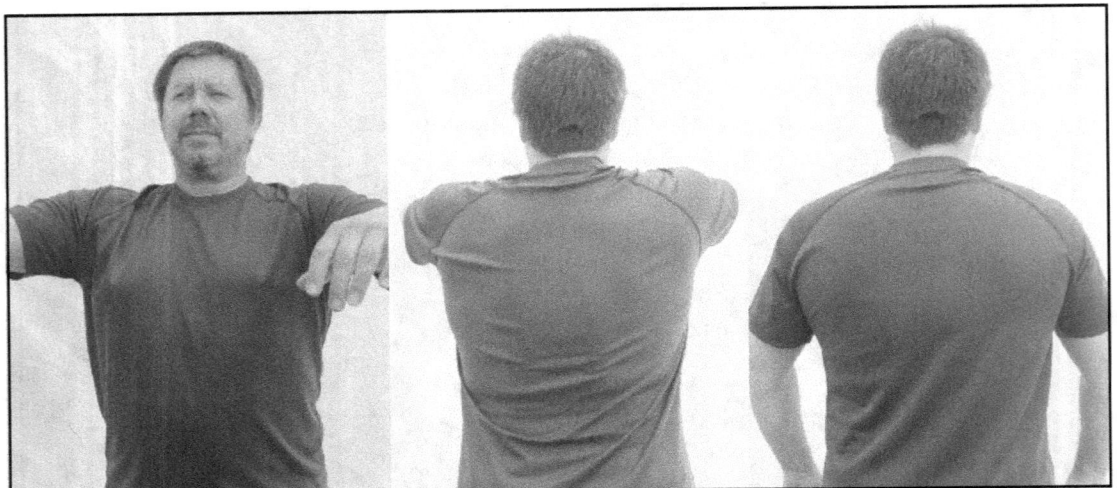

UPPER BODY

So let us look at the chest first. Get back into the Circular Breathing again this time be more aware of your chest movement. Remember, open is expansion, not tension! Closing means sinking and relaxing the chest as much as you can and letting the back round out.

Once you have that feeling, add it in to your movement. Let's stick with the lift hands exercise we just did. Run through the exercise again. This time feel how on the lift, as you inhale, the ribcage can expand and the chest open out. You can exaggerate the movement at first to get the feel. One way to do this is to squeeze the shoulder blades together a little on the lift. Now, on the exhale, as the hands lower, allow the chest to relax, sink and close, as the shoulder blades open out. As I mentioned, exaggerate at first, over time the movement will become more subtle. This is "open and close" in the chest and can be applied to every inhale/ exhale. Let's look at the same concept in the hands.

THE HANDS

Let's work one hand first to get the idea. Hold the hand in front of you, thumb up. To open, push the centre of the palm forward a little, letting the fingers open out. Although the fingers open, be sure not to tense them. Now close the palm. The fingers curl in slightly, the palm is concave. I think of this as the way a magician palms a coin. Once you have the basic idea, work both hands together. This movement has the effect of working one of the main acupuncture points in the body, called Lao Gong. So let us know take a look at the other main points worked by the Eight Brocades.

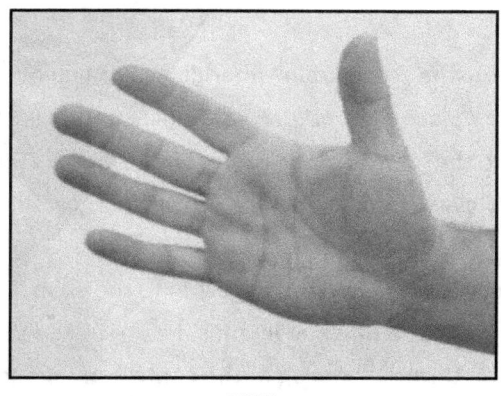
OPEN

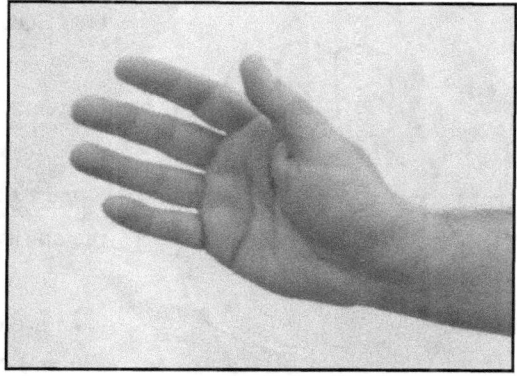
CLOSE

ACUPUNCTURE POINTS

As we mentioned previously, according to TCM, energy travels through the meridians. Certain points are situated along each meridian, known as pressure points or acupoints. There are 20 meridians, 12 of them main ones, and hundreds of points along them. For the purposes of the Eight Brocades, we will look at five major points. It is not necessary to know about these points in order to do the basic exercise movement but knowledge of them will help when it comes to the internal aspects. Let's work from the head down.

BAI HUI

Point 20 on the Governor Vessel meridian. This point is known as the *Hundred Convergences*, a reference to the six yang meridians and the Governor Vessel channel, all of which meet at this point. In the practice of acupuncture, Bai Hui is used generally to "clear the senses." Specific disharmonies that it can resolve include headaches, tinnitus and sinus problems.

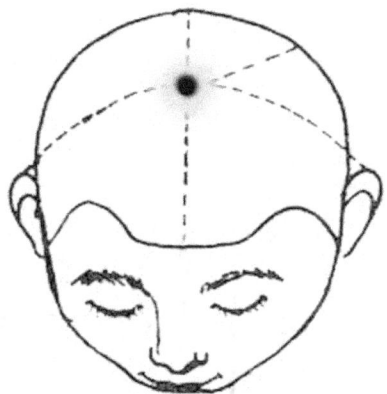

Bai Hui is situated on the crown of the head. To find it, rest the tips of your thumbs at the apex of your ears. Reach your middle fingers up to touch one another, at the crown of your head. You may be able to fine-tune your location by feeling for a spot that feels particularly "alive."

In esoteric terms, Bai Hui is regarded as the gate between Human and Heaven and in other traditions is also known as the Crown Chakra.

LAO GONG

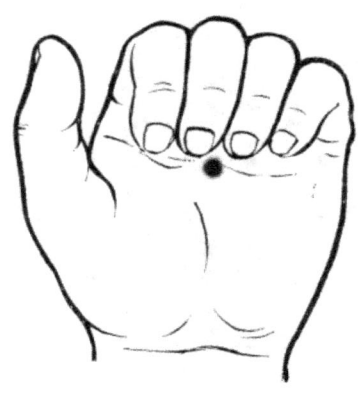

Point 8 on the Pericardium meridian. This point is known as the *Palace Of Labour*, a reference, perhaps, to the fact that the pericardium protects the heart (the *Emperor*). Its classical acupuncture use include calming the spirit and resolving fatigue.

To locate this point, curl the fingers in to the palm. LG is where the tip of the ring finger lands (i.e., between the 3rd and 4th metacarpal bones). In the context of qigong, LG is often used to "emit energy" during healing work.

THE DANTIANS

The Dantians are situated on the front of the body. They are also called *Elixir Fields* or *Energy Centres* and correspond with the main Chakras of other traditions.

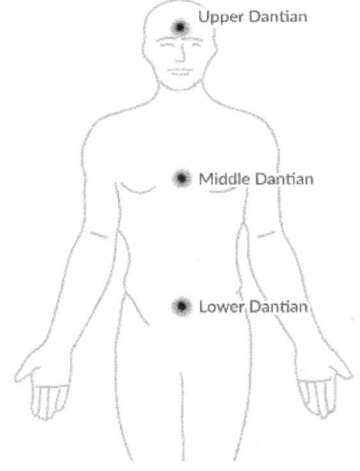

The Lower Dantian is seen as the main energy storage centre of the body. In more physical terms it is our centre of gravity. To find the LD, go three finger widths below your belly button, and think 2-3 finger widths into your abdomen, straight toward your back.

Many qigong practices involve focusing on the LD as part of the sinking / energy storage process.

THE MING-MEN

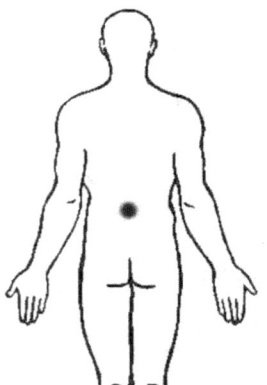

The Ming-men, or *Gate of Vitality*, is another energy centre, situated between the kidneys, at the level of the second lumbar vertebrae.

In TCM terms it serves many functions, including powering the digestive system, developing sexual energy and regulating the kidneys. To find it, take your hands to the spot on your back opposite the belly button. This area is often used as part of the open and close process to "pump" energy up the spine / GV channel.

YONG QUAN

Yong Quan, or *Bubbling Well*, is situated in the centre of the sole of the foot. It is Point 1 on the kidney meridian.

This point lies in the depression that appears when the toes are curled. It is between the second and third metatarsals, about one third of the distance between the base of the second toe and the heel. If you press with your thumb you should feel the point quite easily.

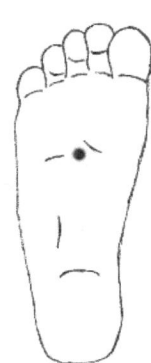

In acu-terms the point is used to revive. It is also seen as our earth connection which, when opened, allows energy to flow from the soles of the feet up to the crown of the head. It can open and close in much the same way as the Lao Gong points in the hand, particularly if you are practicing bare-foot.

FEELING THE ENERGY

All this talk of energy may seem somewhat vague. However, there is a very simple exercise we can practice to help us feel the body's natural energy. It uses the open and close method in the palms we described earlier.

Hold the hands in front of the chest, as though you are holding a large ball. The palms face inwards. Exhale and move the hands apart, inhale and bring the inwards, until they are almost touching. As you inhale, the palms "close". On the exhale, as the hands come together, the palms open. If you practice this open/close exercise for a while you may get a sensation of heat or energy between the palms. Later on we can use this heat in our massage and other therapies. For now, it is enough to be aware of the movement during the exercises.

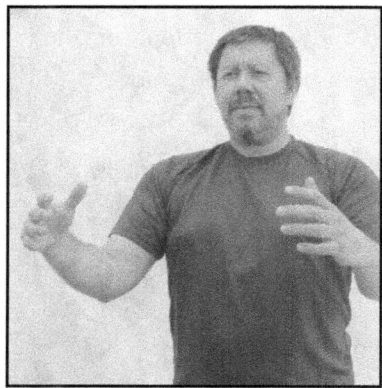
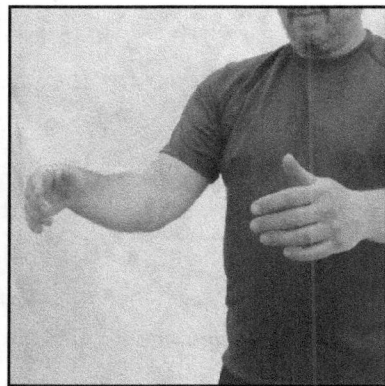
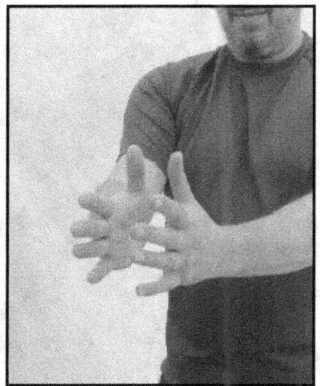

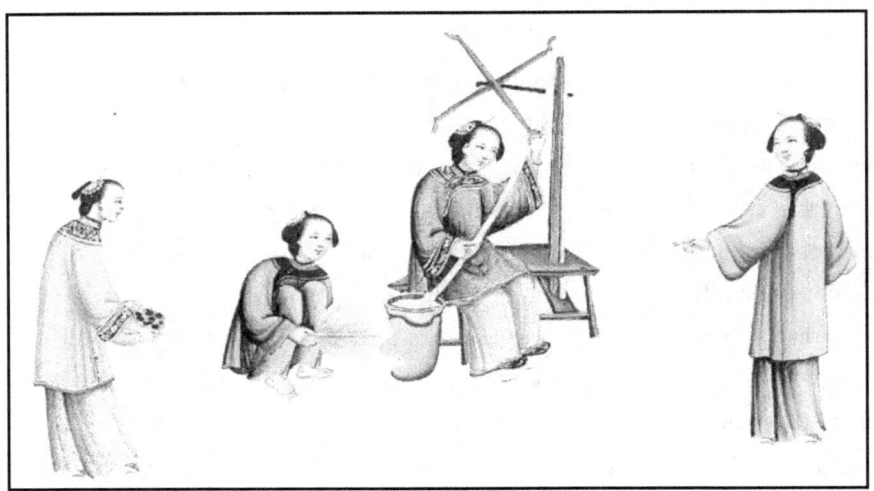

SILK REELING

Another aspect of the "movement within movement" principle in Chinese arts is what is known as *Chan Su Jin*, or Silk Reeling. This refers to coiling motions within the exercises. The idea comes from the motion of someone pulling a thread of silk. Their movement has to be soft and continuous, so that the silk doesn't break. The pulling movement is spiral, so as not to apply direct pressure to the thin thread.

Applied to the body, it can be practiced in larger or more subtle movements and is driven internally rather than by tense muscles. It works the whole system; nerves, tendons, muscle, bone and meridians.

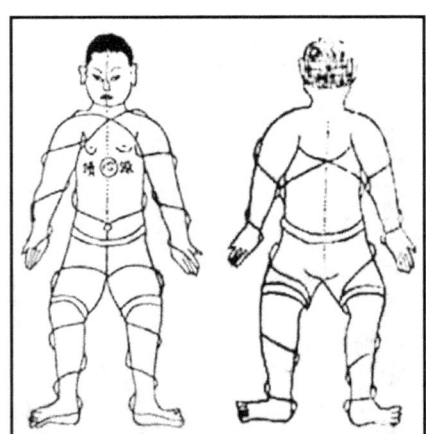

It is entirely possible to practice silk reeling exercises as a form of qigong. In fact, many martial arts use them as a form of body preparation for the practitioner, as they help re-pattern our movement away from local tension and into the area of using wave or spiral motion to drive what we do. Traditionally the preserve of martial arts, this kind of work is now becoming more popular and prominent amongst athletes, dancers and sports people. It can be an an involved and complex practice, but let's look at a basic method that will get you into thinking about spirals.

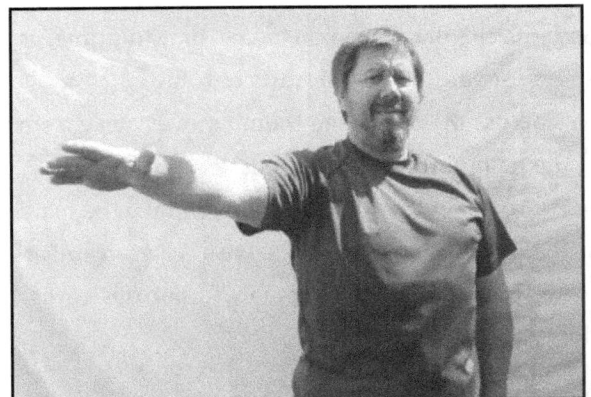 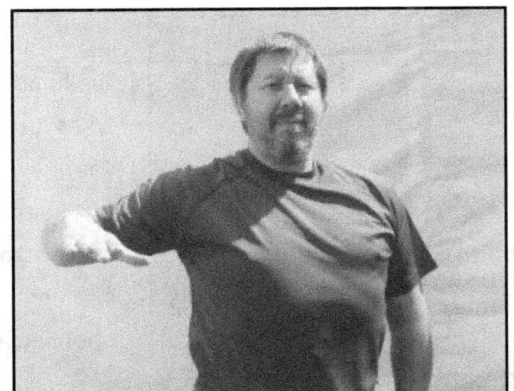

Hold your right hand out to the side with the palm down. Keeping the shoulder relaxed, circle the hand forward, then across the chest to the left side of the body.

From there, complete the circle back to the start position. Repeat, so that your are making a counter-clockwise circle with the hand at chest height.

Movements like this are often called *Polishing the Mirror* in Chinese arts, for obvious reasons. You can also think of it as a form of "wax on, wax, off" if you remember the Karate Kid! Repeat with the left hand.

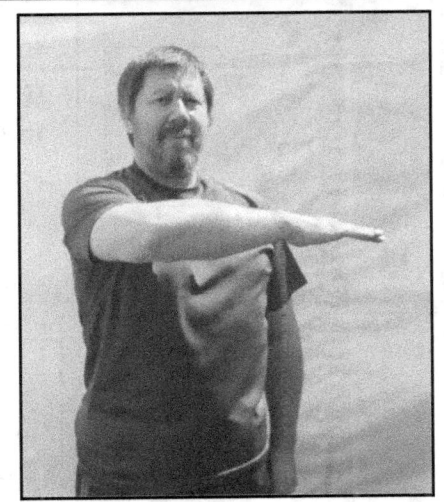

The key is to make a smooth, flowing circular movement in a flat pane. The body is not involved at this stage, just the arm. Keep the breathing natural and easy.

Even just doing a basic movement like this can help with the shoulders and begin to loosen tense muscles. Now, let's add in some spiral

Start with the right hand in the same position, except this time the palm is facing forwards. Once again, check to make sure the shoulder is relaxed.

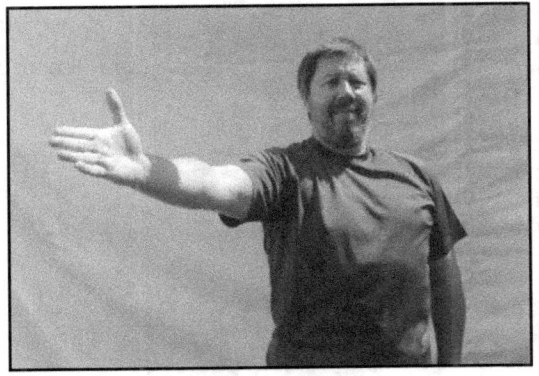

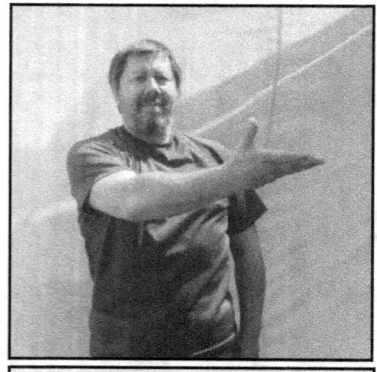

Start the same circular movement again, only this time, as the hand moves forward, the palm starts to rotate.

So as it moves across the chest, the thumb moves away from you, turning the palm through 90 degrees.

Keeping the torso and shoulders square on, take the hand as far across to the left as you can. If you wish, you can add an opening of the shoulders in at this point, as per our earlier open and close movement.

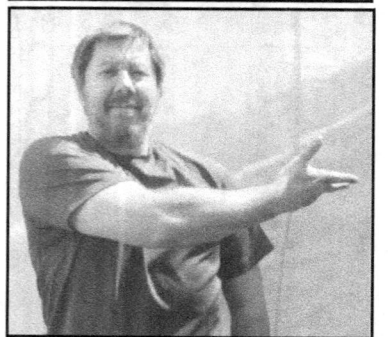

Once the hand has gone as far to the left as it can, you start on the return half of the circle. Once again, the palm rotates as it moves across the body. The thumb now rotates towards you as the hand makes a kind of scooping motion back across the chest.

This type of movement is often called *Teacups* in qigong. You circle the hands whilst keeping the palms flat - as though you have a teacup in the hand and do not wish to spill any tea!

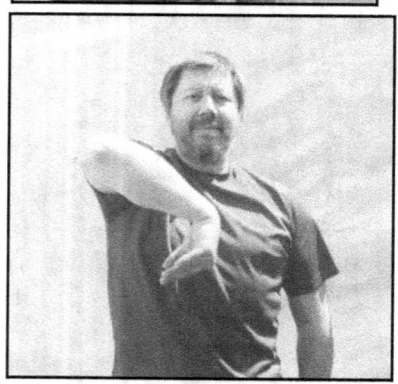

As the hand returns back out to the start position, the rotation continues. The thumb now rotates backwards in order to bring the palm back to its forward facing position.

The point now is that within that simple circle, we have a spiraling or coiling motion. Try on both sides!

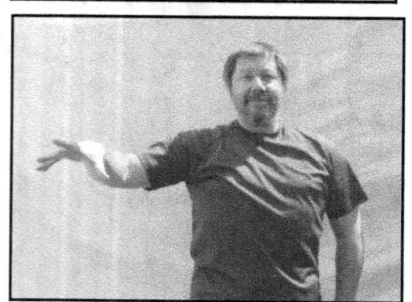

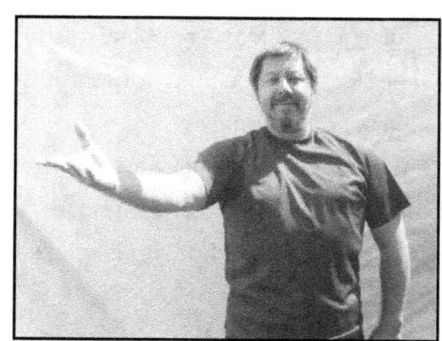

GROUNDING

The final principle we will look at is grounding. This is another very common concept amongst Chinese arts. In short, grounding is the principle of establishing a strong connection, or root, with the ground. In martial art terms, we see this in strong, low stances, which provide a stable platform for the hands to work. In less combative terms, grounding can be seen as the process of connecting us back to our centre and our root.

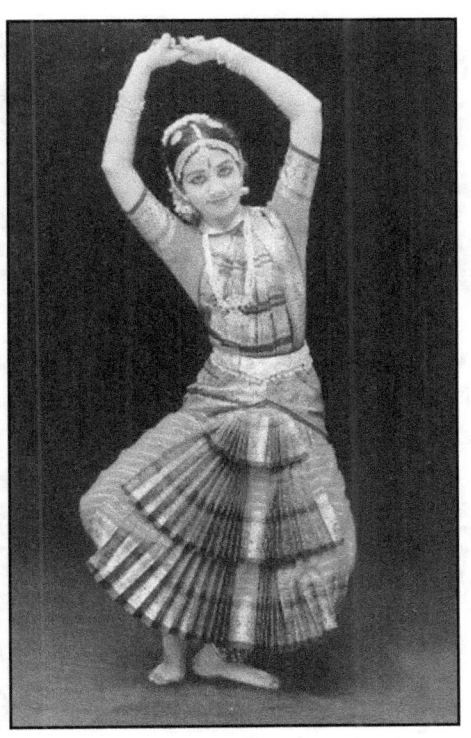

The principle can be felt very easily. The next time you start to feel stressed or upset, remove yourself from the situation, if possible, and spend a couple of minutes in basic horse stance, practicing circular breathing. Allow all the tension in your body to drop, sink your stance down into the soles of the feet. Become aware of the Lower Dantian. Focus the mind on that point, slow the breathing, still the mind. Hopefully that will be enough to "centre" you and help stop negative emotions from lifting you up and carrying you off into anger!

It is interesting to note how so many indigenous cultures have dance forms that involve barefoot contact with the ground and stamping movements. Slavic health practices include cold water dousing, where you stand barefoot outside and slowly pour cold water over the crown of your head. Today, it is very easy to lose our natural contact with the earth. The principle of grounding can help us to re-connect and bring us back in control of our emotional and psychological state.

All of these different aspects can be added to even the most basic of exercises. Gradually work each of them in as you become more familiar with the Eight Brocade movements. Do not neglect them, as these fundamentals are what takes qigong beyond just a "fancy stretch" and into the realms of internal exercise.

So, having covered all the basics, let's begin!

CHAPTER THREE
THE EIGHT BROCADES

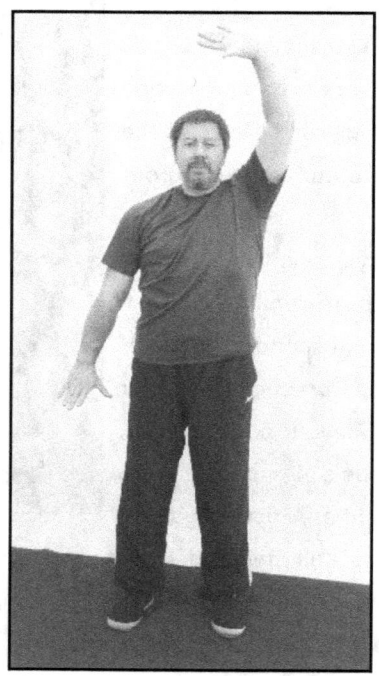

THE EIGHT BROCADES

We will now go through each of the eight movements in turn. We will describe the basic movement, what it is for, and also add in some details on the breathing and open and close aspects.

The main thing at first is to get all the external aspects of each exercise correct. The movements are quite straightforward but, as we have already seen, doing even a simple movement with perfect posture is quite a challenge.

I recommend you run through the basic "routine" of each exercise a few times. Get the feel for each. When you feel comfortable with it, move on to the next one. Once you have done all eight, put aside a little time and run through the whole sequence. Unlike Tai Chi there are no real connecting movements between the exercises. So after each, you can just come back to normal resting position between each exercise and pause for a little.

In terms of repetitions, at first run through each movement around six times. As you become more used to the exercises and as you add in the extra layers, you can increase up to a dozen or even twenty or more reps. Some advise doing 24 reps of each movement to get maximum benefit, though it also depends how much time you have available.

If you only have a little time free, do not neglect your practice! It is better to do few movements regularly than do the complete routine once a month!

While The Eight Brocades can be practiced by people in most conditions, if you do have a particular ailment, always check with your Doctor first. If, at any time during the routine you feel discomfort or pain, stop immediately and get yourself checked over. The movements are slow but can place pressure on legs and back, so always move with care.

Some movements involve twisting and bending at the waist. Take care if you have back issues - always work slowly. When bending, keep the back as straight as you can. Always lead the straightening up movements with the head. If you feel at all dizzy when bending, come out of the exercise immediately and sit quietly for a few minutes.

Take all aspects step by step, especially the breathing. Qigong and similar exercises are designed to be long term healing methods, not "quick fix" fitness routines.

Above all, try to perform the movements with "mindfulness." As mentioned before, this is what separates this type of work from "conventional" fitness methods. If you do, I'm sure you will discover benefits far beyond what maybe apparent from such seemingly slow and simple moves.

We also include a preparation and finish movement. These are not strictly part of the sequence but give a nice "ease in and ease out" bookend to the routine.

PREPARATION

Opening

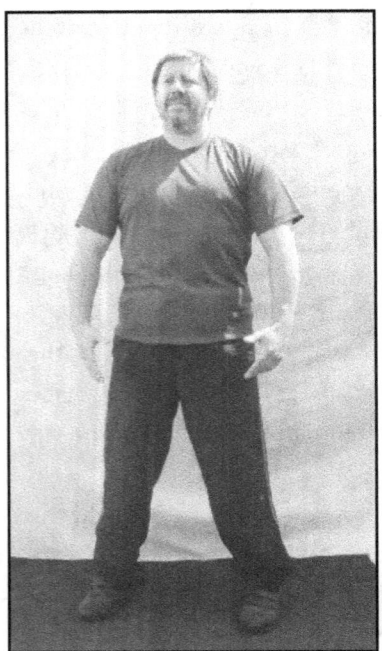 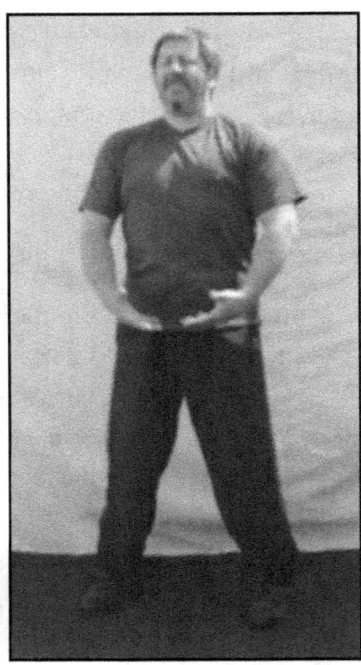 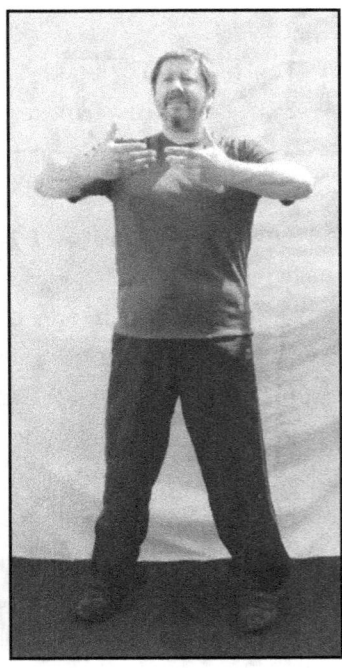

Stand in normal stance. Hold the hands at the sides. Keep the arms slightly rounded, chest and shoulders relaxed. Go into Circular Breathing and begin to slow the breath.

When you are ready, begin an inhale and bring the hands in to the lower Dantian.

Lift the hands in time with the breathing. As the hands lift, the thumbs turn in, rotating the palms towards you.

BENEFITS

This exercise is a standard "opening" movement in qigong. The aim is to prepare the body and mind for the routine to come. As you run through the movements try and still the mind and relax the muscles into the standing posture. In internal terms, this movement is designed to open the acupoints Bai Hui, Lao Gong and Yong Quan and bring awareness into the Dantians.

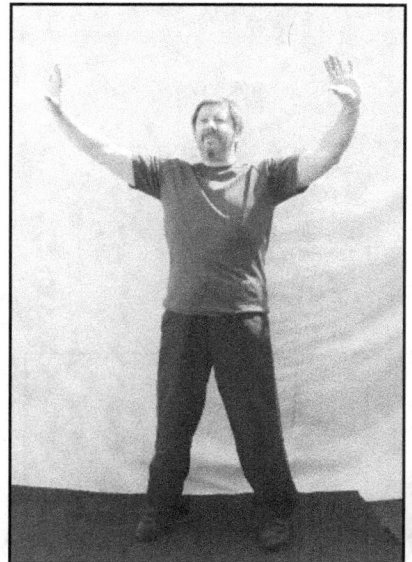 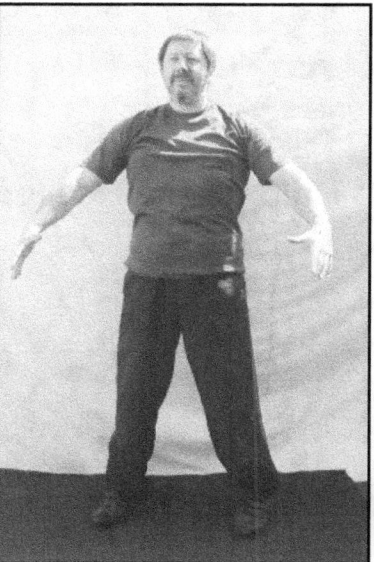 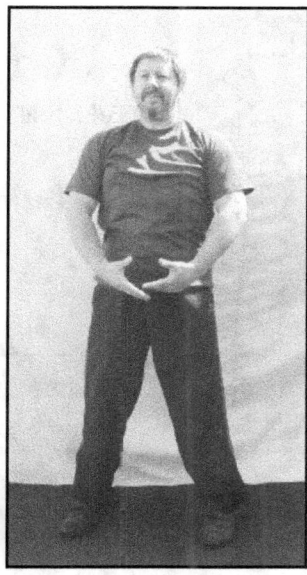

Take the hands up past the face, then open them out to the sides.
The inhale finishes at the upper point of the movement.

Begin the exhale as the hands start to circle down. Remember to keep the arms slightly rounded.

Complete the inhale as the hands return to the Lower Dantian.
Note again how the palms rotate back to their original position.

BREATHING

Inhale as the hands raise, exhale as they lower.

OPEN & CLOSE

Palms close at the lower position and open as they circle up.
Chest opens on the inhale, relaxes on the exhale.

SILK REELING

The hands and arms spiral on the upward movement.
They make a "scooping" type circle on the downward movement.

VISUALISATION

Feel the main points opening, from crown of head to soles of the feet. Energy rises from the Lower Dantian up the spine and out into the palms.

Simply Flow - The Eight Brocades

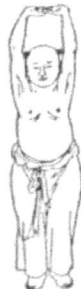

MOVEMENT ONE

Two Hands Hold up the Heavens

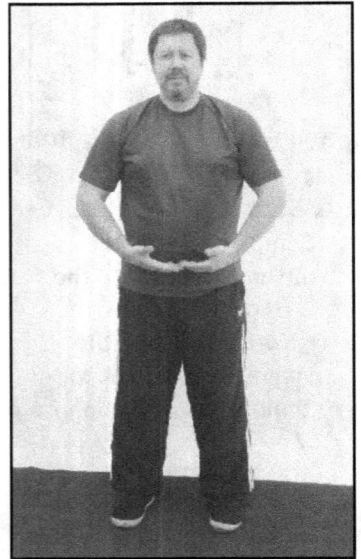
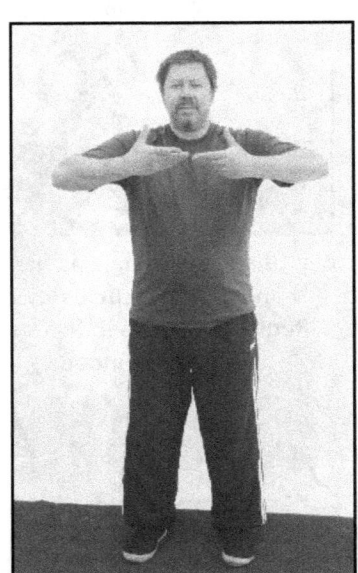
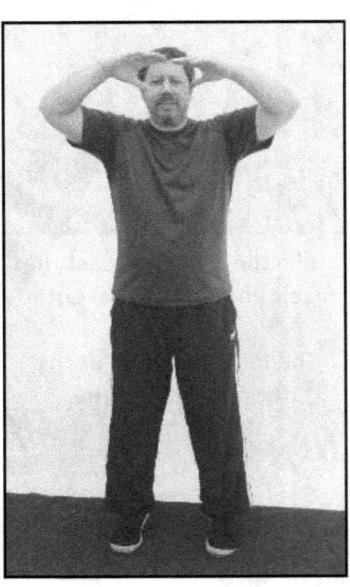

Stand in normal stance. Hold the hands at the Dantian, palms up, fingers almost touching. Check your shoulders are relaxed. Knees are straight but not locked.

Inhale as you begin to raise the hands. Make sure that as the hands lift, the shoulders remain relaxed.

The palms rotate as the hands come up. The thumbs turn towards you, so that as the hands reach face height, the palms are facing down.

BENEFITS

Balances the energy flow in the Triple Warmer meridian (*sanjiao*). This is primarily associated with the endocrine system and our fight or flight response. An unhealthy Triple Warmer can result in issues such as ADD, chronic fatigue, anxiety and panic attacks as well as insomnia and tinnitus. Practicing this qigong will benefit all these conditions.

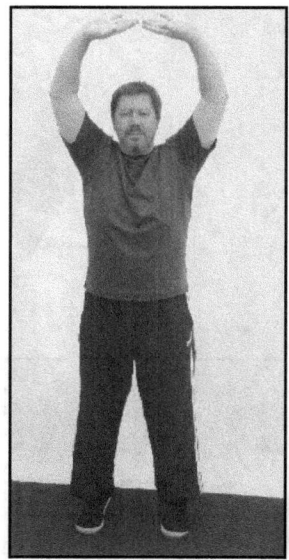 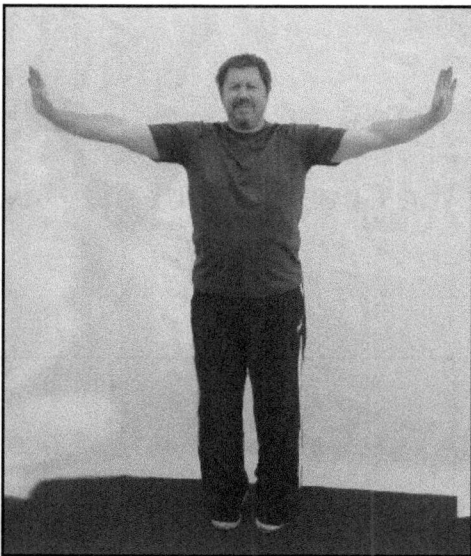 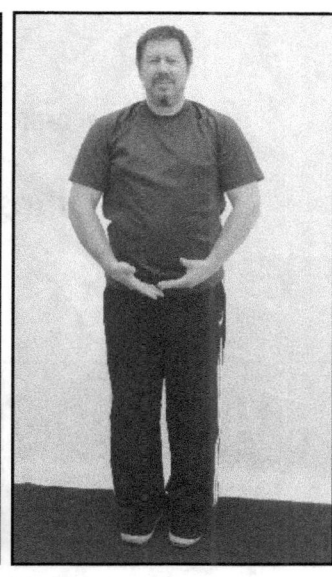

Continue rotating the palms until they face upward again.
Push upwards, with the fingers facing in.
If your balance is okay, you can also raise up onto the toes.

Now bring the hands down and out to the sides as you lower the heels back down. Exhale.

As the exhale finishes, the hands return to the start position.

BREATHING
Exhale as the hands lower, inhale as they raise up.

OPEN & CLOSE
Palms close at the lower position and open as they push up.
Chest opens on the inhale, relaxes on the exhale.

SILK REELING
The hands and arms spiral on the upward movement.
They make a "scooping" type circle on the downward movement.

VISUALISATION
The hands push up to "touch the sky". The spine lengthens.

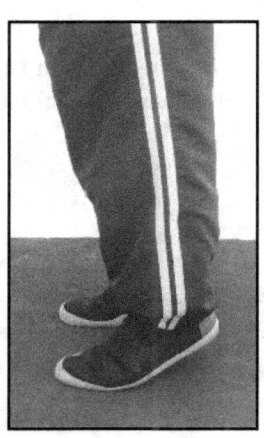

The heel raise.

Simply Flow - The Eight Brocades

左右開弓似射鵰

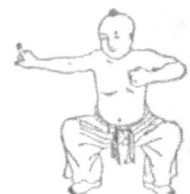

MOVEMENT TWO

Pulling the Bow to Shoot the Hawk

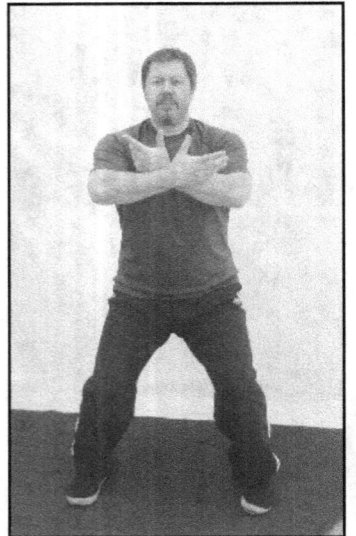 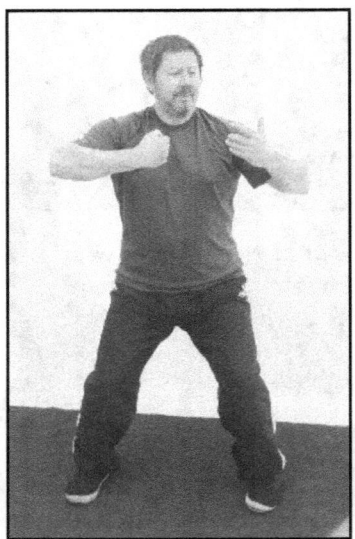 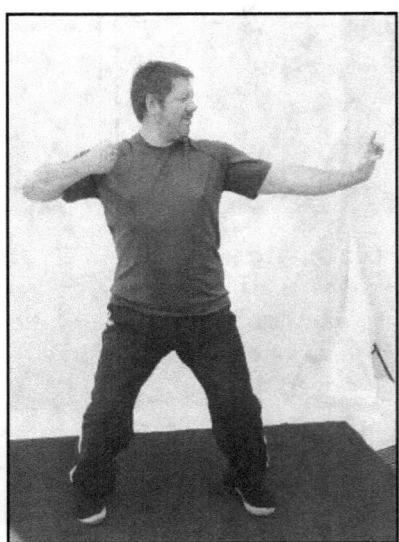

Stand in horse stance. Cross the hands at chest height, with the right hand on the outside.	The right hands makes a fist and begins to pull back to the side. Start an inhale. The left hand begins forming a "tiger claw" (see inset photo)	The right fist pulls back completely. The left hand pushes out to the left. The head turns to gaze beyond the left hand.

BENEFITS

Balances and replenishes the kidney meridian. Strengthens your root through the low horse stance. Works on strengthening and realigning the lower back muscles and the spine.

Simply Flow - The Eight Brocades

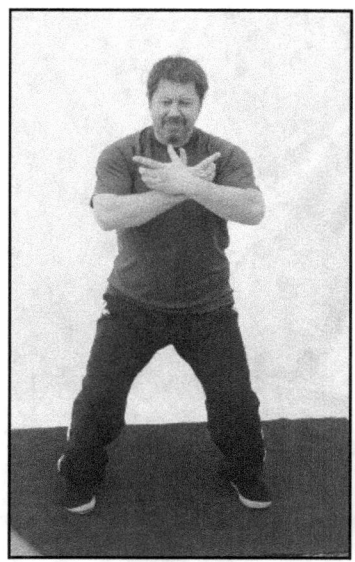 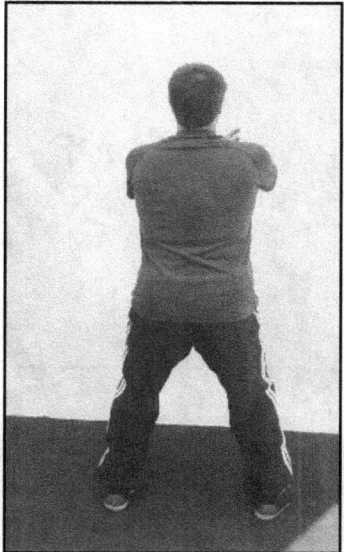 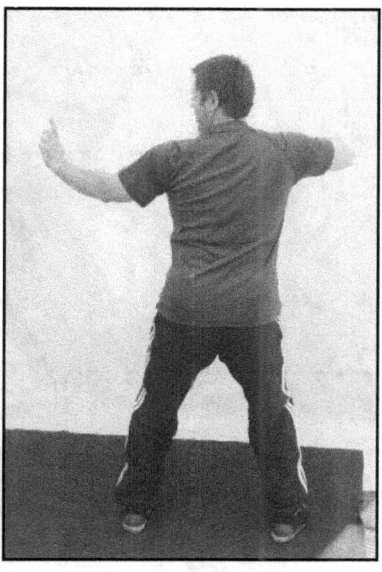

Exhale as you "release the arrow" and cross the hands once more. This time the left hand is on the outside.	Repeat the movement, this time it is the right hand pulling back. Keep the weight sinking down into the stance.	Remember to turn the head to look out beyond the pushing hand. Imagine you are looking at the "target".

BREATHING

Inhale as the hands open, exhale as they return to the chest.

OPEN & CLOSE

Palms close at the pull and open as the arrow is released.
Chest opens on the inhale, relaxes on the exhale.

SILK REELING

Both arms spiral slightly on the push and pull movement.
They scoop as they return to cross over the chest.

VISUALISATION

Imagine you are pulling a bowstring, so there is a little tension in the hands. As the arrow is "fired" the hands relax. Gaze out each side to the "target."

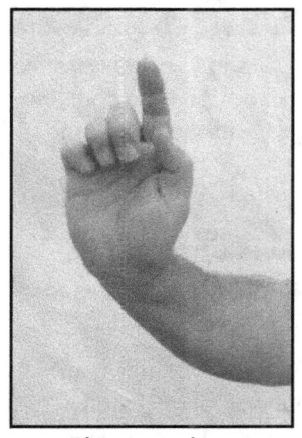

The tiger claw.

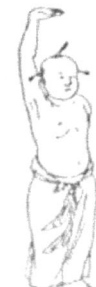

MOVEMENT THREE

Separating Heaven and Earth

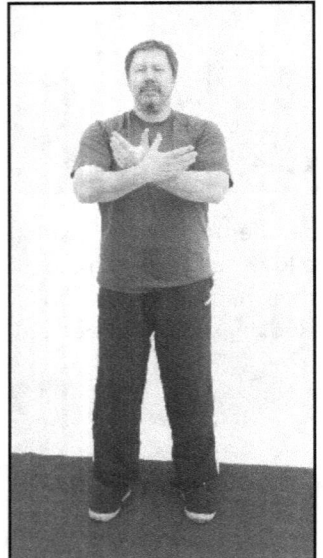
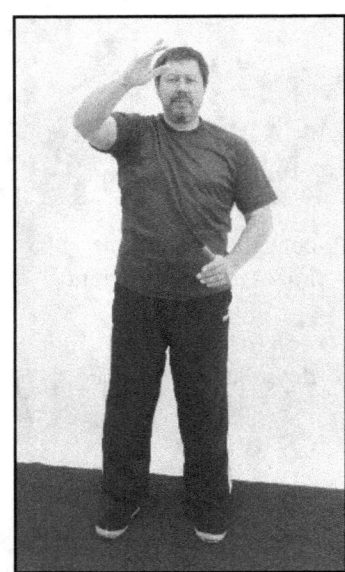
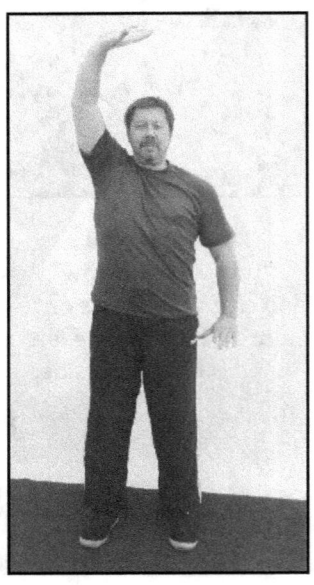

Stand in normal stance. Hands cross at chest level, with the right hand to the outside. Keep shoulders relaxed and arms rounded. Start an inhale.

Begin to raise the right hand. The left hand lowers. Note how the palms rotate as the hands move.

As the inhale ends, the right hand is pushing up and the left hand is pushing down. Note the position of the fingers. Upper fingers point to the side, lower fingers point forward.

BENEFITS
Balances the spleen and stomach meridians and also regulates the liver and gall bladder. The abdominal cavity follows the motion of the alternate and opposing pull, creating a "massaging effect" on the spleen and stomach. Simultaneously, it will adjust both sides of the rib cage, passageway of the liver and gall bladder meridians.

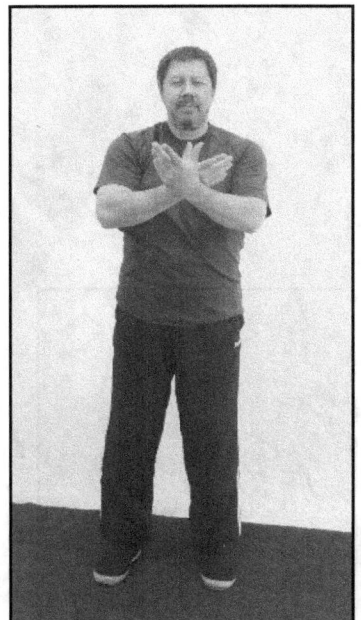 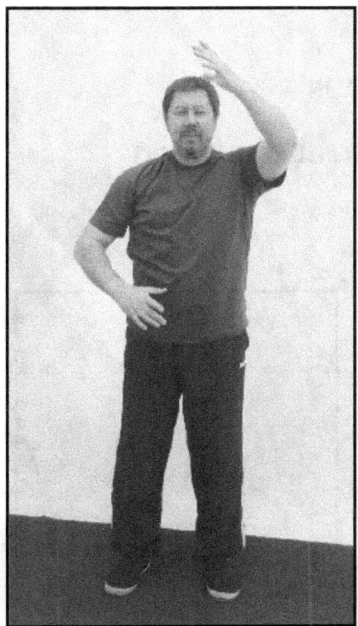 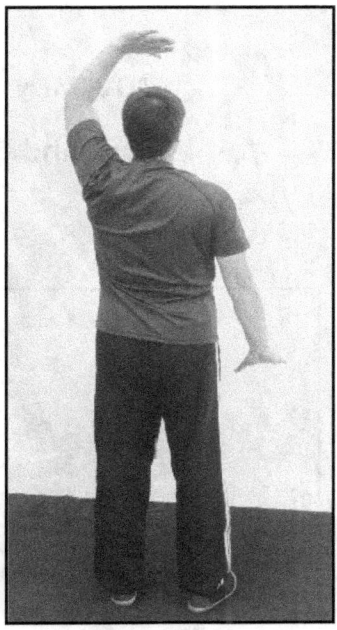

Exhale as the hands now return to the start position. Once again, the palms rotate. Note that this time, the left hand is on the outside.

Repeat the movement, this time with the left hand pushing up and the right hand pushing down.

Note again the position of the fingers. Keep the body square on as you push up and down.

BREATHING
Exhale as the hands cross, inhale as they push up and down.

OPEN & CLOSE
Palms close at the crossing and open on the push.
The shoulders open as the hands cross.

SILK REELING
Both arms spiral as they move up and down.

VISUALISATION
Imagine you are trying to push on the ceiling and floor at the same time. Feel the sides open and stretch.

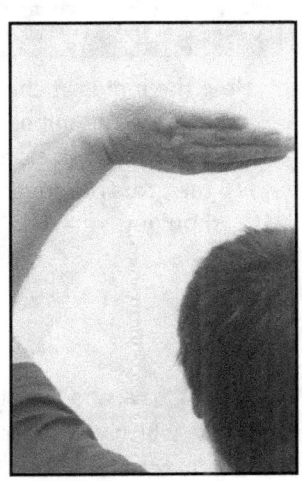

The upper hand

五勞七傷往後瞧

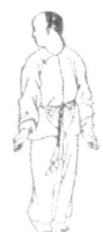

MOVEMENT FOUR

Turn and Gaze at the Moon

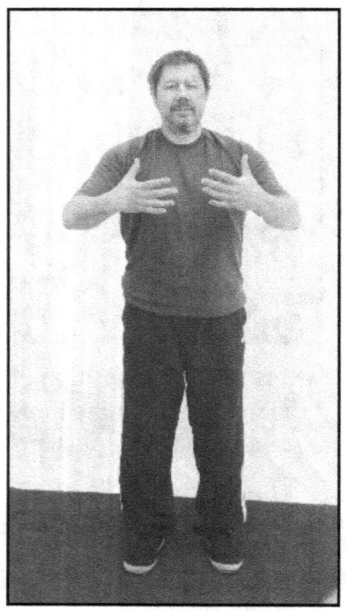
Hold the hands at chest height in the upper Zhan Zhuang position. Keep the arms rounded and shoulders relaxed.

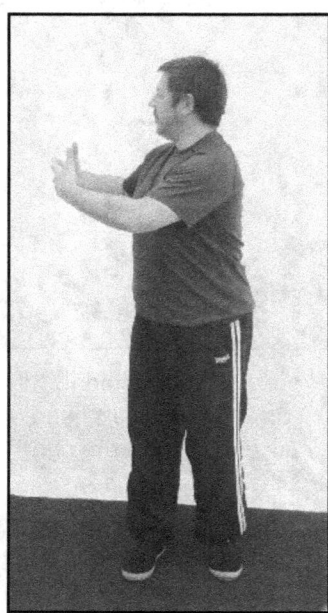
Inhale and turn the waist to the right. The hands do not move yet, they just follow the rotation of the trunk. Keep the knees relaxed.

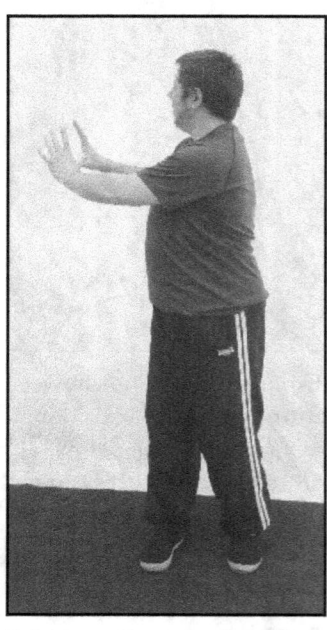
Exhale and rotate the palms outwards, pushing the hands away from the body. Keep the elbows slightly bent.

BENEFITS

By looking back and focusing the eyes to the back, we twist our spinal cord to enhance the role of the yang, which will help prevent diseases and external damage. The second part of the movement is the arm rotation. The arm has six meridians. This movement of the arms will help activate the yin and yang in these meridians.

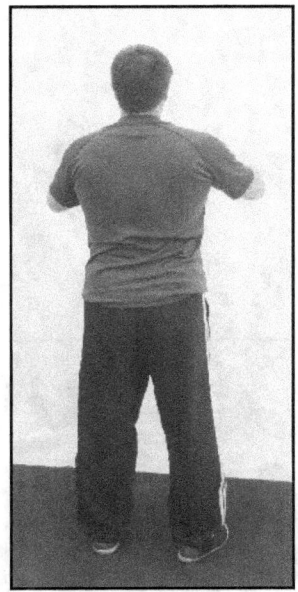 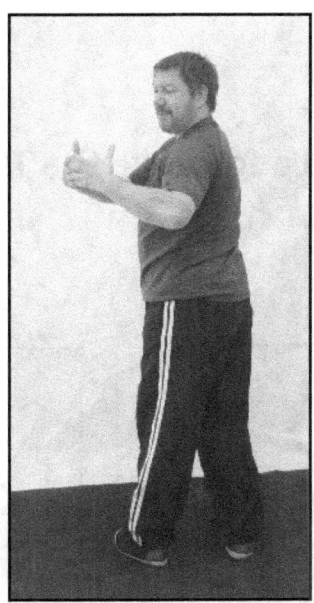 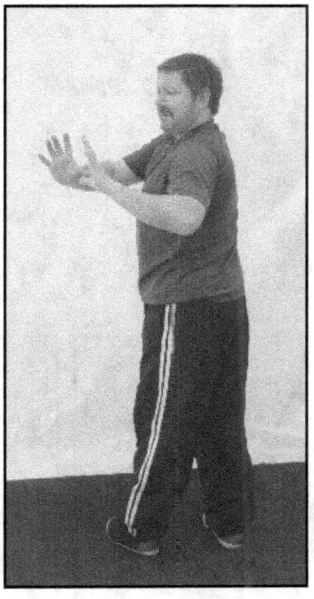

Inhale as the palms turn back in to face the body. The torso returns to the centre.

Keep the inhale going and turn until you are facing to the left.

Exhale as you push out to the left. Be sure to keep the body upright and try and turn the waist as far as you can on each side.

BREATHING
Inhale on the body turn, exhale on the push.

OPEN & CLOSE
Palms close at the centre and open on the push.
The chest opens on the inhale, the shoulders open on the push.

SILK REELING
Both arms spiral on the push.

VISUALISATION
Imagine you are pushing something away from you. As you do, the eyes "gaze" to the point you are pushing to.

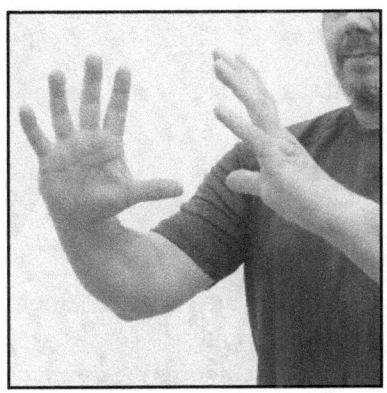

The push

Simply Flow - The Eight Brocades

摇頭擺尾 去心火

MOVEMENT FIVE

Sway the Head and Shake the Tail

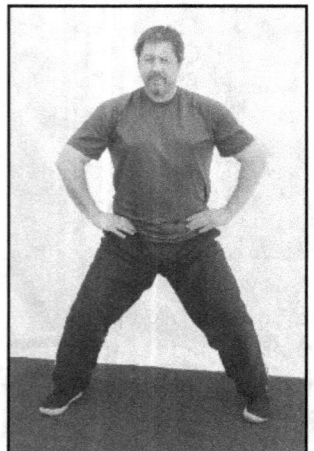
Stand in wide horse stance with the hands on your hips.

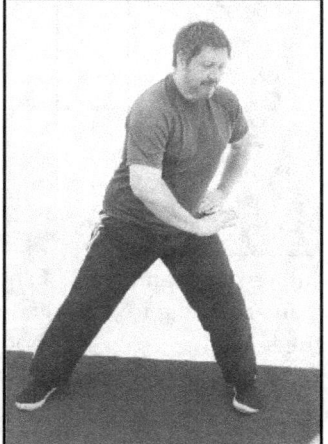
Start an inhale and turn the body until you are facing to your left, shifting the weight a little into your left leg.

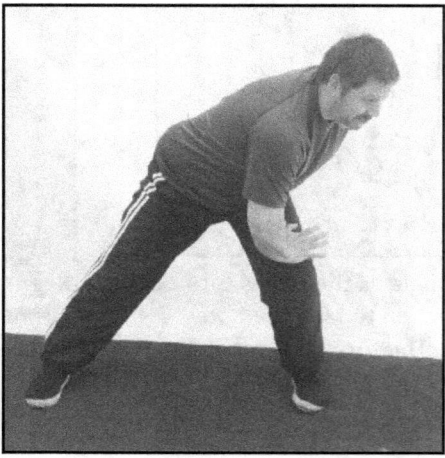
Exhale as you lean forward to place the right hand onto the top of the left knee.

BENEFITS
The horse stance will strengthen and condition the legs. Bending and turning at the waist strengthens and stretches the hip, abdominal, and lower back muscles.
This exercise reduces the excess of heart fire and strengthens the energy of the kidneys.

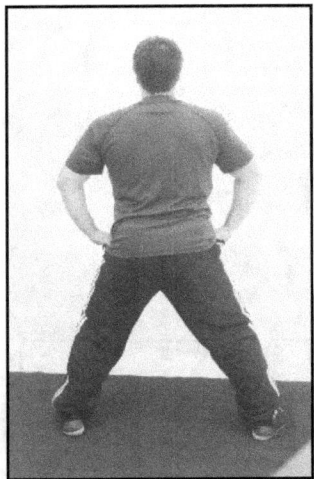 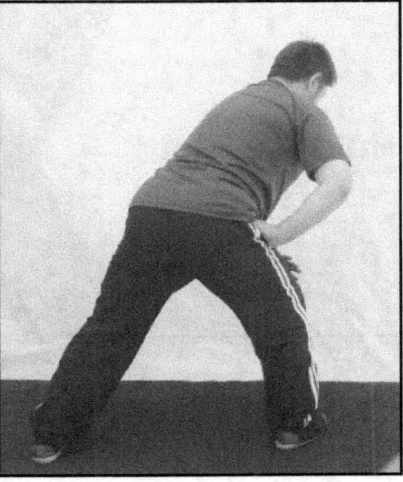 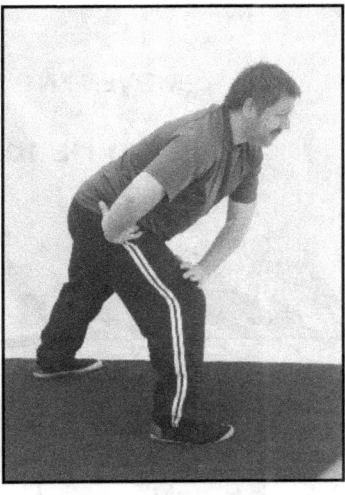

Inhale and return to the start position, shifting the weight back into the centre. When you straighten the body, lead the movement with the head.

Repeat the movement to the right. Left hand now goes to the right knee.

When you lean, be sure to keep the lower back straight. Push the hips back a little and the head forward.

BREATHING
Inhale on the turn, exhale on the lean.

OPEN & CLOSE
Palms close at the turn and open on the knees.
The chest opens on the inhale. The Ming Men opens on the lean.

SILK REELING
The torso can twist a little once you are used to the movement.

VISUALISATION
Project out from the crown of the head on the lean.
Imagine energy projecting from Lao Gong into the knee.

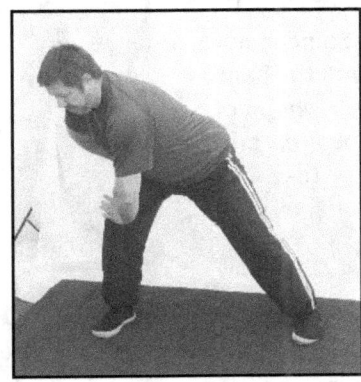

Simply Flow - The Eight Brocades

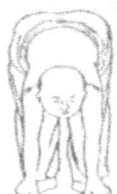

MOVEMENT SIX

Two Hands Hold the Feet

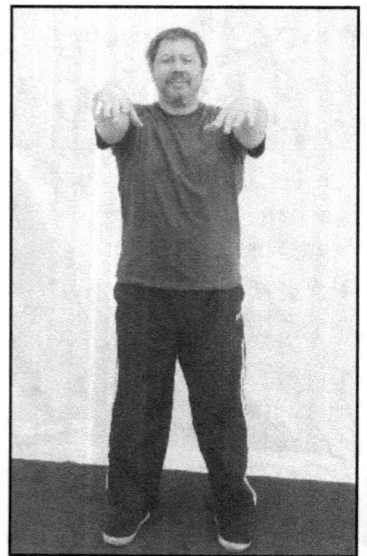
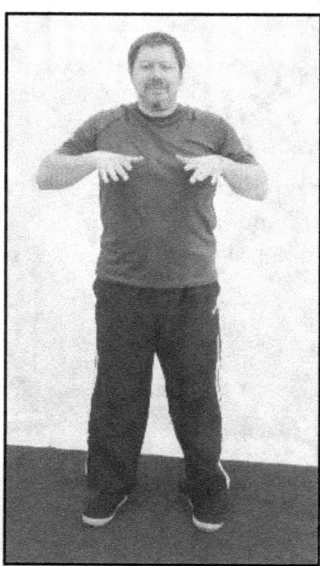
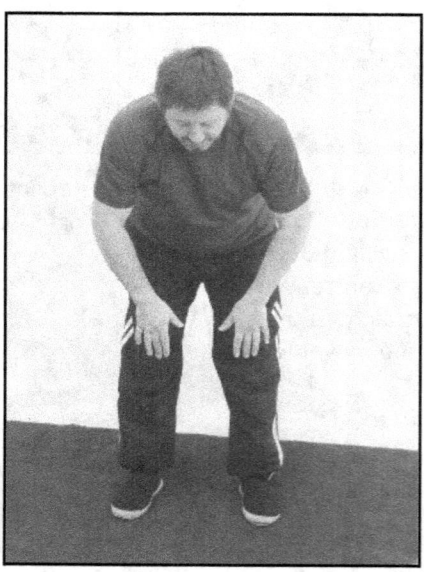

Stand in normal stance with the hands held out at shoulder height.
The arms are slightly bent.
Take an in breath.

Start to exhale as you bring the hands in and down.

Bend at the waist as the hands move down towards the feet.

BENEFITS

Creates a vertical massaging effect and stretch on the back. This will exercise and stimulate the spine and the meridians in the back. Through inhaling and exhaling, the abdominal cavity, waist and back muscles and the meridians will be stimulated. Strengthens kidneys and adrenal glands.

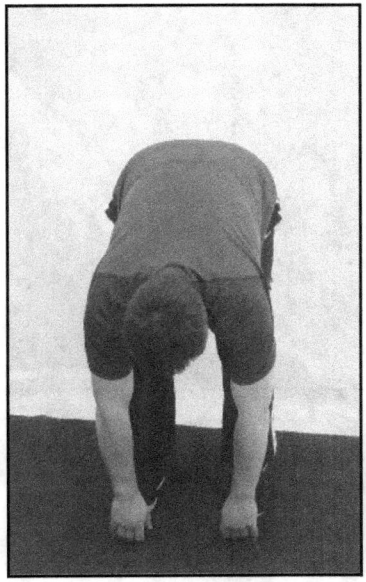 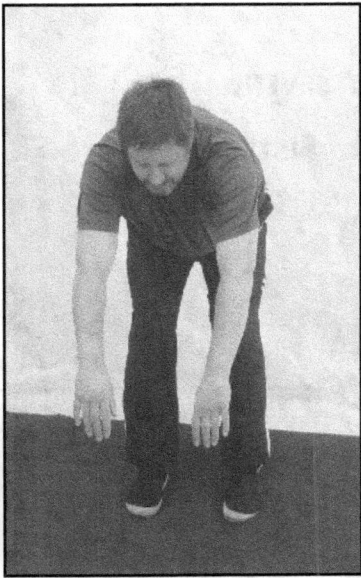 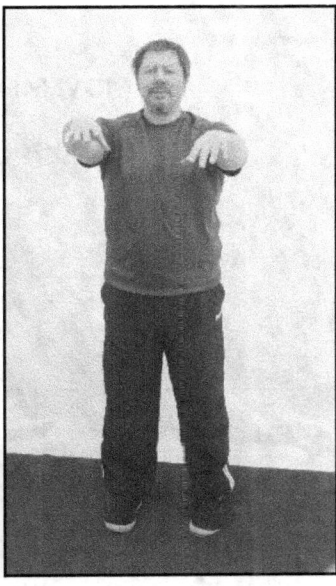

As the exhale ends reach down as far as you can. If you are able you can grab the toes and hold for a second.

Start to inhale as you straighten, bringing the hands forward and up.

The inhale finishes as the hands return to the start position.

BREATHING
Inhale on the lift, exhale on the bend

OPEN & CLOSE
Palms open as they reach the toes, close as the hands lift.
The chest opens on the inhale. The Ming Men opens on the bend.

SILK REELING
The arms spiral slightly on the lift.

VISUALISATION
Lengthen out the lower back on the bend. Be sure to lead with the head when you straighten up. Keep the knees straight for more of a stretch in the legs.

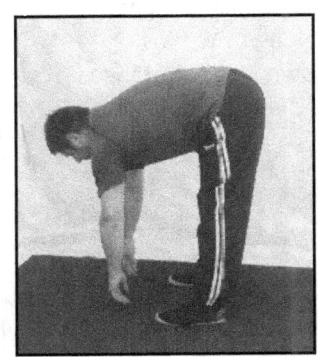

MOVEMENT SEVEN

Clench the Fists and Glare Fiercely

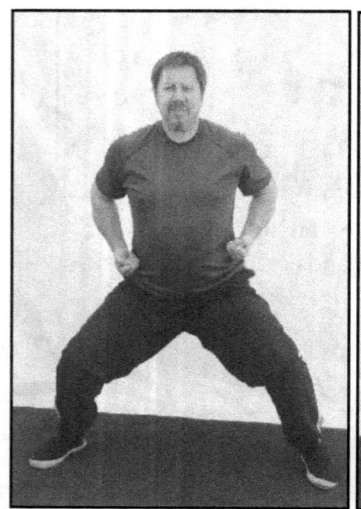
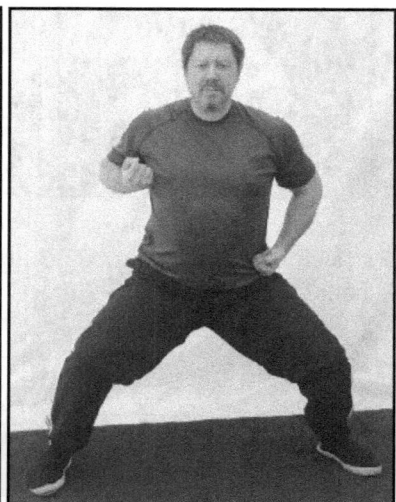
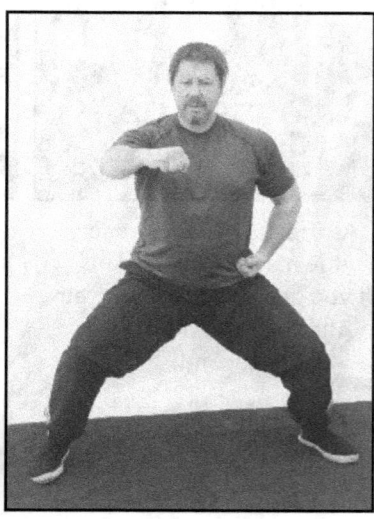

Stand in wide horse stance. Clench the fists and hold them at the hips. Sink down into the stance, keep the spine straight.

Inhale as you bring the right fist up to chest height.

Exhale and push the fist forward. As the hand moves out, it rotates from palm up to palm down.

BENEFITS

Squatting down exercises the leg muscles. Angry and tense feelings are vented, released, and dispelled. Helps stimulate and revitalise the liver. Improves overall strength and determination.

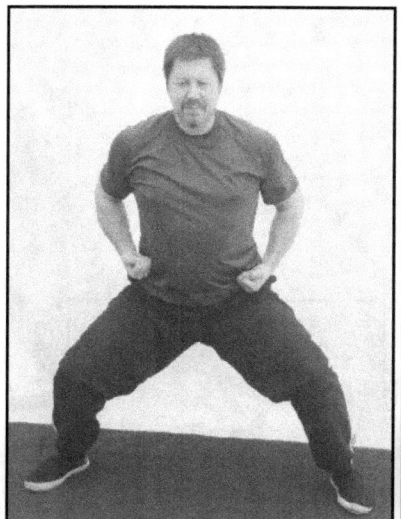 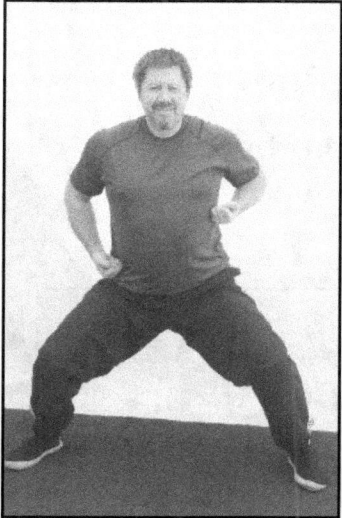 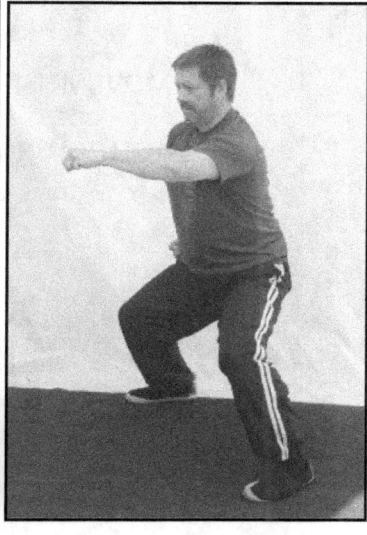

Inhale as you bring the fist back in and down to the hip again.
The palm rotates upward as it comes back to the chest.

Repeat the same movement with the left fist. The body can rise a little as the fist lifts and sink a little on the punch.

When you push out, do not totally straighten the arm, keep it slightly bent.
The forearm stays parallel to the floor.

BREATHING
Inhale on the return, exhale on the punch.

OPEN & CLOSE
Palms open on the punch (inside the fist!)
The chest opens on the inhale. The back opens on the punch.
Feet open as the weight sinks down.

SILK REELING
The arms spiral on the pull back and punch

VISUALISATION
Project a firm gaze out beyond the fist. Imagine there is some resistance to the fist pushing forward and also that you are pulling something back on the return.

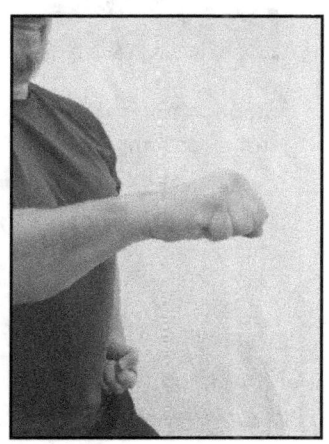

The fist

Simply Flow - The Eight Brocades

我後七顛百病消

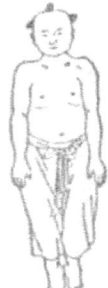

MOVEMENT EIGHT

Bouncing on the Toes

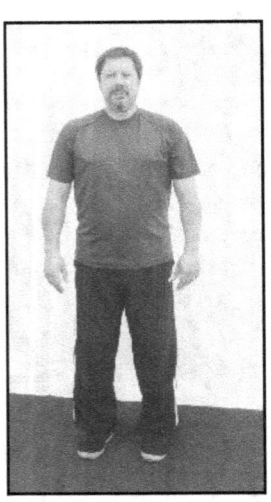

Stand in normal stance with arms hanging at the sides.

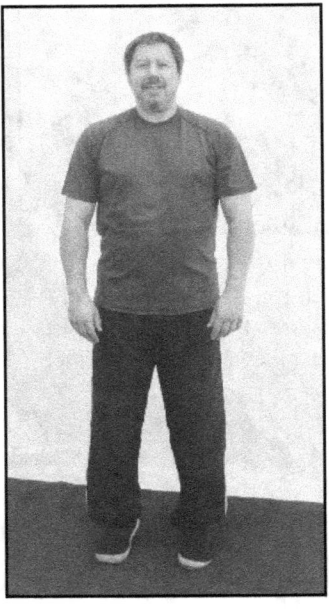

Inhale and lift up on the toes. Keep the body straight.

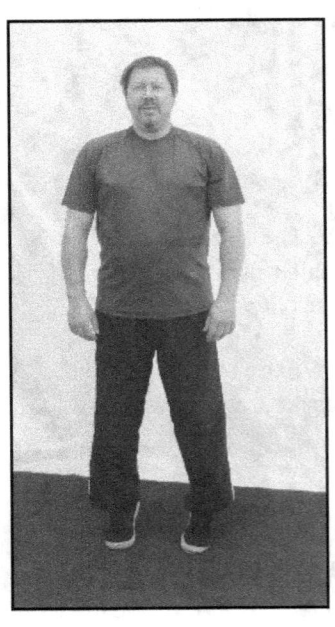

Exhale and drop the weight back down.

BENEFITS

Gives a good calf workout. Stimulates the lymph to flow. Bouncing, vibrating, or shaking, the internal organs is considered to have positive health benefits in many Chinese qigong systems. Also excellent for your spine, nervous system, and sense of balance.

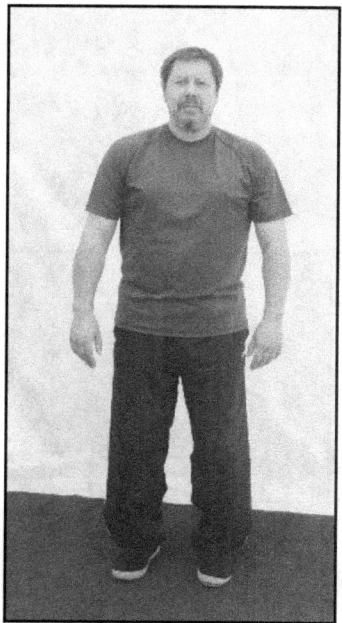

When you impact the floor, keep the whole body relaxed. Allow the shock to travel through the whole body.

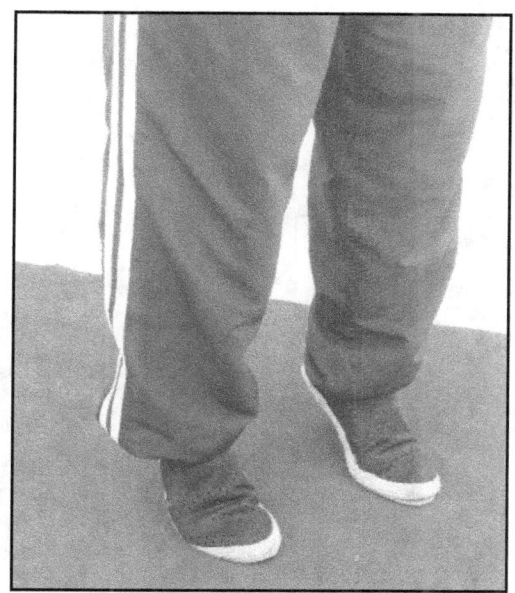

When you lift up on the toes, see if you can "close" the Young Quan points.

BREATHING

Inhale on the lift, exhale on the drop. The exhale can be quite sharp.

OPEN & CLOSE

The chest opens on the inhale. The back opens on the drop.
Feet close on the lift, open as the weight drops.

SILK REELING

Once you get the feel, allow the impact to travel through the body in a wave type motion.

VISUALISATION

Try and keep the whole body relaxed but do not let the structure collapse. Be especially careful with the jaw, teeth and tongue on the drop!
You can hold the lift position for a little if you like.

FINISH MOVEMENT

Closing and Grounding

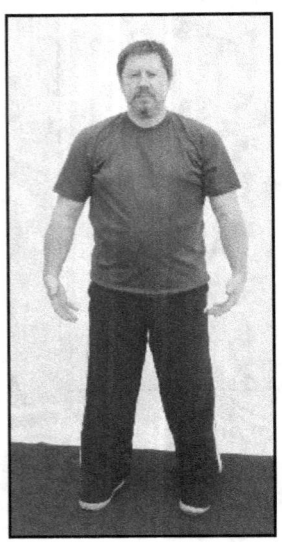 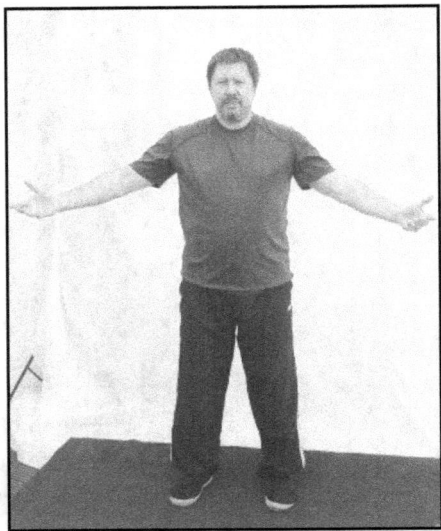 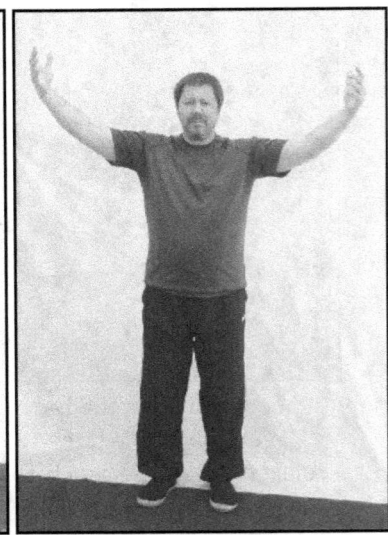

Stand in normal stance with arms held at the sides.
The palms face upwards.

Inhale and start to raise the hands out to the sides. The palms still face upwards.

Keeping the shoulders relaxed, raise the hands above the head.

BENEFITS

This movement is designed to cool the body and mind down and help centre the energy back at the Lower Dantian. It has a powerful calming effect and is very much a "grounding" exercise.

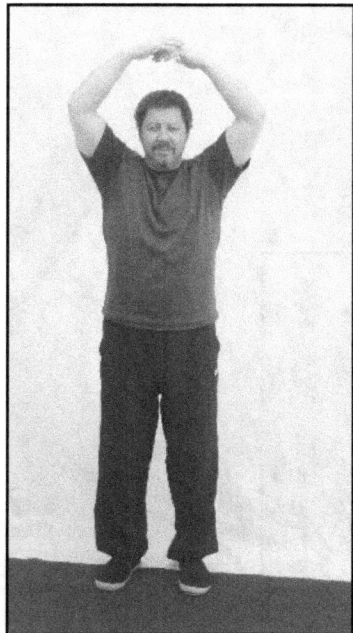 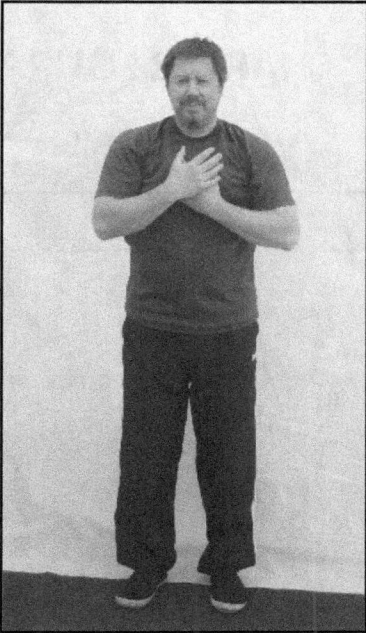 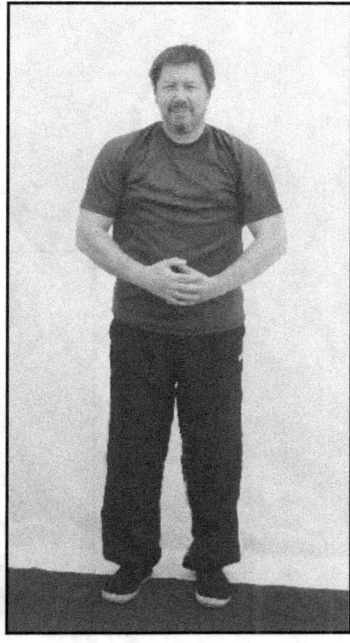

As the inhale finishes the hands are positioned just above the crown of the head.	Exhale and bring the hands directly down the front of the body, palms turned inward. The hands should be an inch or so from the body	Repeat the movement and to finish, rest the hands on the body at the Dantian. Close the eyes and focus on the breathing for a few minutes.

BREATHING
Inhale on the raise, exhale on the lower.

OPEN & CLOSE
The chest opens on the inhale. The back opens on the exhale.
Palms open on the raise, close on the lower. Ditto for the feet.

SILK REELING
Arms spiral slightly in the raise and fall.

VISUALISATION
Imagine energy emitting from Lao Gong at the end the exhale. It transfers into Bai Hui at the crown, then into Governor Vessel as the hands move down the body, finally into the lower Dantian. When at rest, let everything relax and sink down into the feet.
Energy rises up the spine on the inhale, sinks down the front on the exhale.

CHAPTER FOUR
VARIATIONS

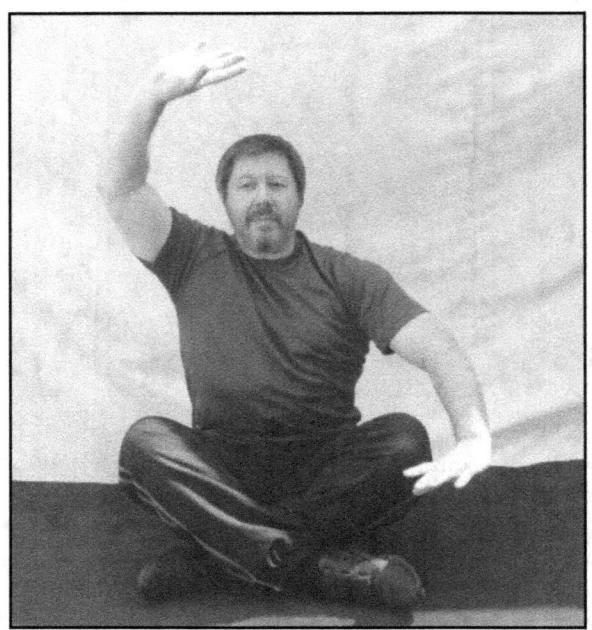

VARIATIONS

As we mentioned before, there are numerous variations of the Eight Brocades, some of which we will show you here. Whatever the variation, it is vital, of course, that the fundamental principles remain in place, however much the outer form varies. The variations are simply the result of the many different schools and teachers who have practiced and developed the exercises over the generations. The variations may also relate to the function of the routine - whether for health, for meditation, or as a body training method for martial arts. Each approach will have its own emphasis.

In the late 1950's, practicing qigong became a political issue in China. The government, via its *People's Sports Press*, published compilations of the major Qigong styles as well as modifications and unification of the various traditional variations. The main focus was on assimilation. "Standard forms" were established for qigong and many martial art practices, such as the 24 Step Taiji Form.

On the one hand this meant that much knowledge was gathered and standardised. So whichever school you went to, you could be sure you were learning exactly the same material. It also meant that form competitions could be judged on a level playing field.

On the downside, standardisation can introduce an element of stasis into an art form. In my view, disciplines such as qigong and martial arts should be as much about personal expression and inner feeling as external "performance". At its worst, this has led to some martial art forms in China becoming little more than glorified gymnastics, which is a great shame.

In the 1970s, the newly standardized Eight Brocades became part of the official sports curriculum of colleges and institutions all over China. If you do a search on Youtube you can find this and many other versions of the exercise, these will also give you some other variation ideas.

Another thing to consider are what we might call "personal variations". This means that we can tailor each exercise to our own personal situation. For example, if you have difficulty standing, it is possible to do most of the exercises sitting down.

Similarly, if you have a major shoulder issue, don't feel you have to do the full range of movement for any of the exercises. If you have back or blood pressure issues, take care on the bending exercises. If you have balance issues there is nothing wrong with using a chair or similar for support.

Remember, while you might feel a little "next day ache" in the legs after working horse stance, none of the exercises should cause sharp pain or major discomfort.

The last variation to consider is the breathing. While we have detailed one set of breath patterns here, do feel free to experiment. Switch the inhale/exhale and see how it feels. Whatever feels most natural for you is usually best.

Separating Heaven and Earth with Turn

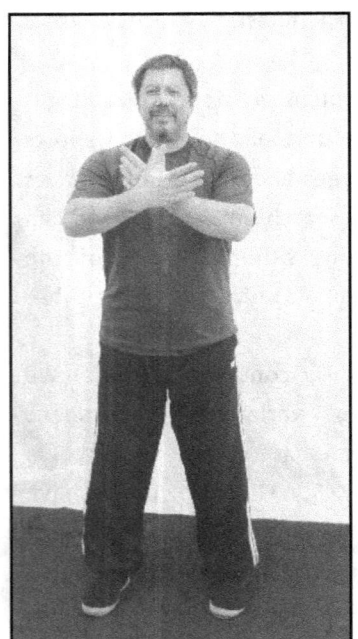 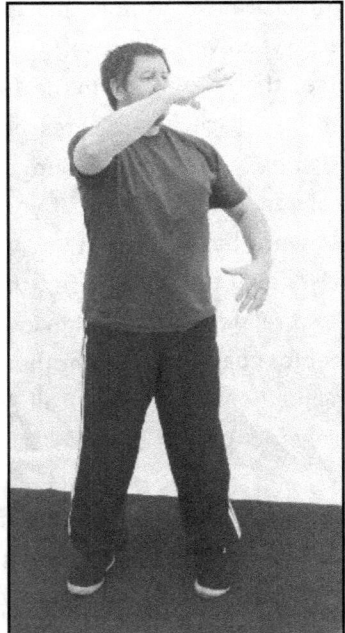 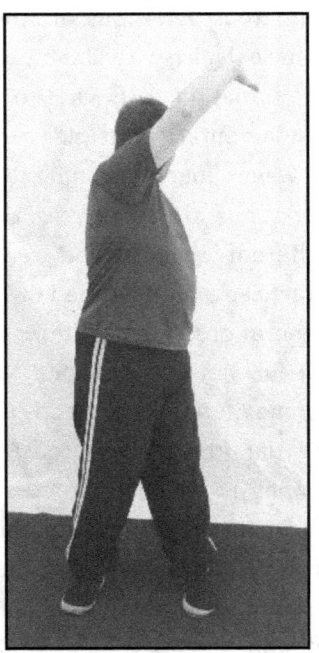

Start in the cross hands position with right hand to the outside. Let's switch the breathing too. Take an inhale.

Start to exhale as you raise the right hand up and take the left hand down. The palms rotate as shown.

As the hands move, the body turns to the left. Twist the waist as far as you can and look down at the floor behind you.

You can use this exercise as a variation of Separate Heaven and Earth or you can think of it as a combination of that exercise and Turn and Gaze at the Moon. So if you are short of time you can do both exercises in one!
Remember, for the extra stretch push the hands up and down at the end of the waist turn.

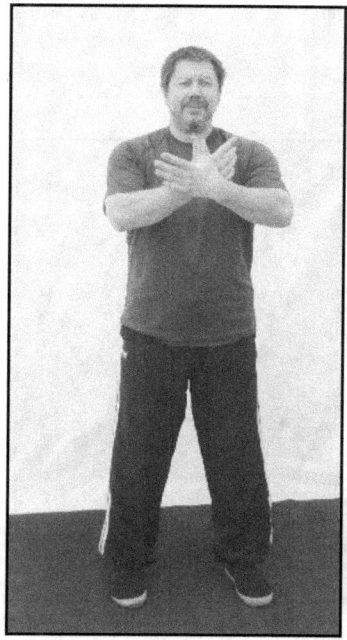 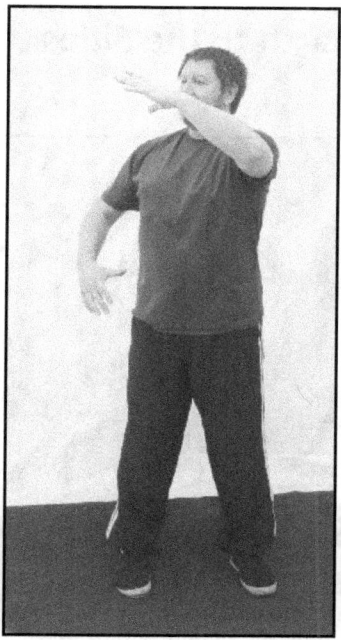 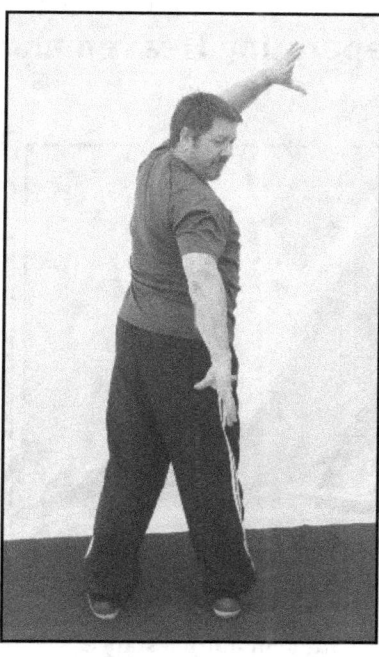

Inhale as you return to the start position.
This time, the left hand is on the outside.

Start to exhale as you repeat the movement, turning the waist to the right.

Note how the gaze is shifted downward at the end of the movement.

There is a very obvious body spiral in this movement but take it easy at first. The feeling should be of lengthening the spine as you twist it. So even though the gaze is down, do not let the head drop, keep it projecting upwards from the crown.

As the body twists, also be aware of the knees. Take care to keep them relaxed and not too fixed in place. We should avoid spiral force going through a locked knee.

If you need to, let the rear heel lift a little and allow the back knee to turn in a touch.

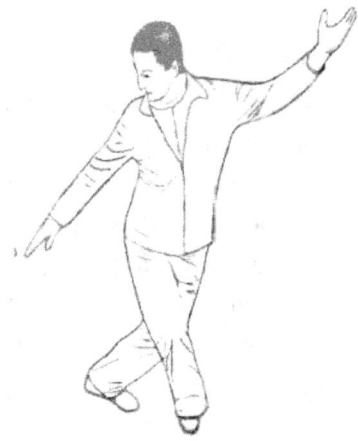

Separating Heaven and Earth to the Sides

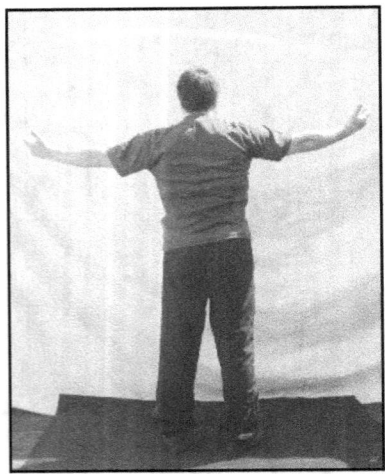 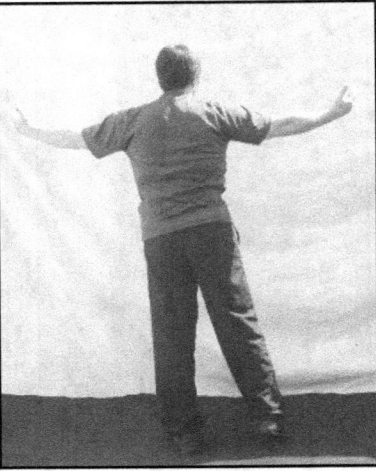 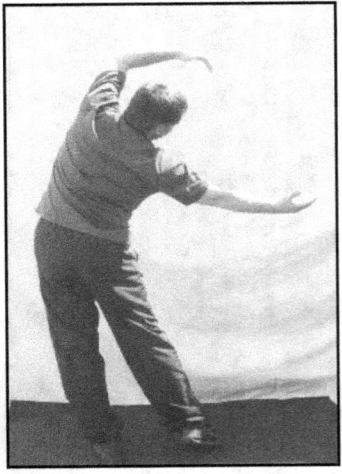

Stand in normal stance.
Bring the hands out to shoulder height, palms up.
Inhale.
Start to shift the weight into the left leg.

Begin an exhale as you raise the right heel. Keep as much weight as you can in the left leg and begin to bend the torso to the right.

Continue the torso bend as you take the left fingers over the head towards the right palm.

    This exercise is also sometimes called *Bend Like a Tree*. This is a common theme in Chinese philosophy. For example, Confucius said: *"The green reed which bends in the wind is stronger than the mighty oak which breaks in a storm."*

    The idea is that in life we must learn to bend and adapt to situations rather than always stand firm and perhaps be broken by them.

    Learning to be flexible on a physical level has a surprisingly strong effect on our mental and emotional health too!

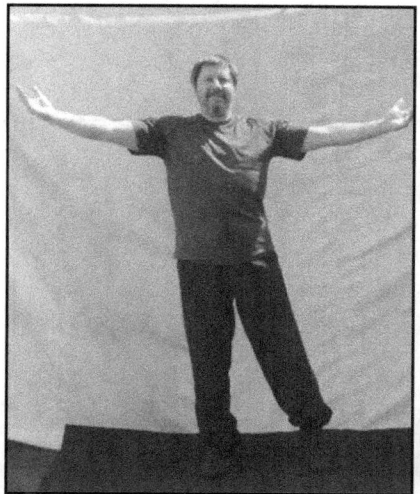 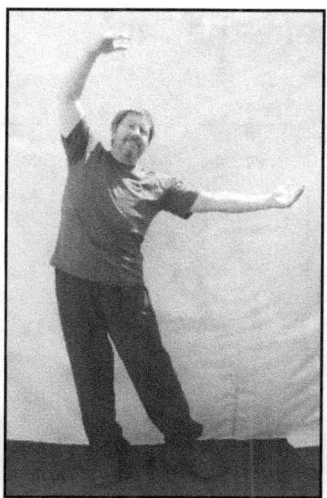 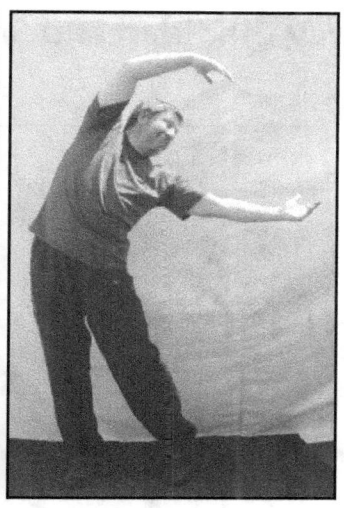

Inhale as you return to the central position.
Be sure to keep the shoulders relaxed throughout.

Now shift the weight into the right leg and raise the left heel.
Begin the exhale.

Continue the bend as before, moving the right fingers towards the left palm.

This is a simple bending motion with little spiraling. However the palms can open/close on the stretch/return.

Be sure to keep the weight as much in the rear leg as possible when you bend. This allows you to "fold" the body more.

For extra stretch, really try and reach across to the extended palm.

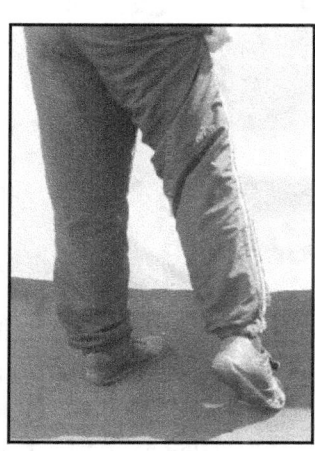

As the weight shifts into the rear foot, the other heel raises off the floor.

Sway the Head and Shake the Tail

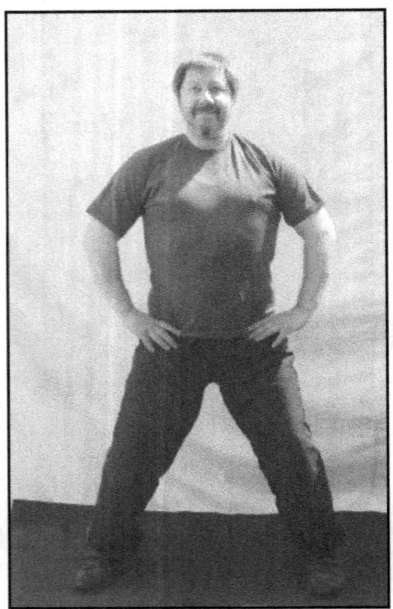
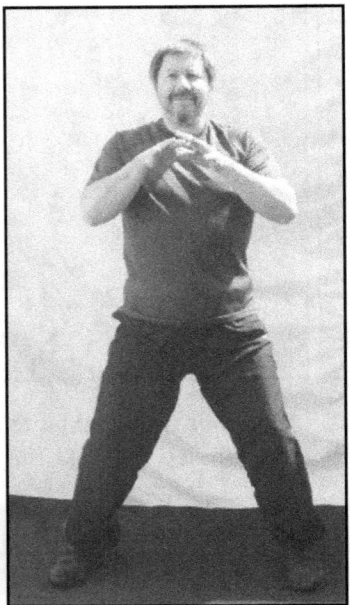
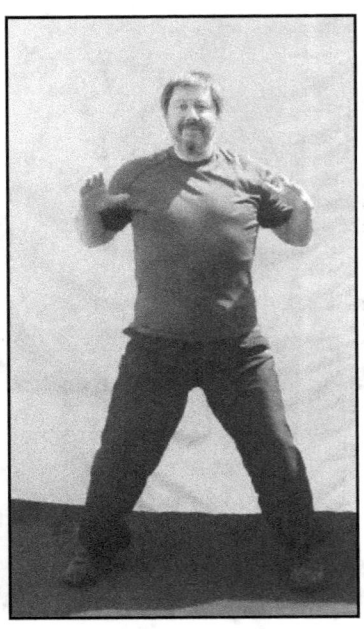

Stand in horse stance with hands on the hips. Start in inhale.

Bring the hands up to chest height, the palms facing down.

As the inhale finishes, draw the hands out to just in front of the shoulders.

This movement is a little similar to the posture *Push* in the Taiji form. The arms make a swimming type motion, you can think of it as a reverse breast stroke!
Sink down into the legs on the forward movement, this will help to shift the hips back.

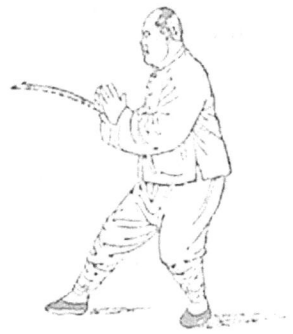

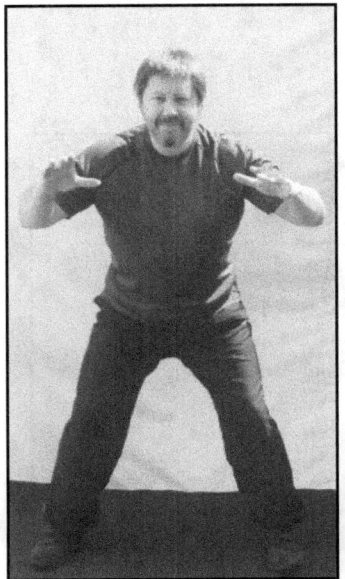 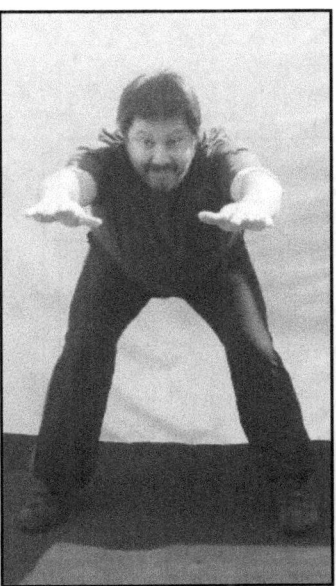 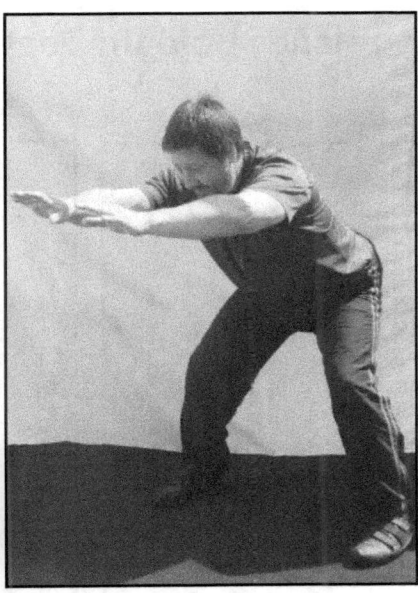

Start an exhale.
The hands now extend forwards. Sink the weight down into the legs.

Stretch the hands out, at the same time push the hips back.
Do not let the head sag.

Make sure you keep the back as straight as possible. The aim is to lengthen the spine.

As with all bending exercises, be sure to keep the lower back straight and lead with the head.

You can also practice this movement as a static stretch. Lean on a chair, or grab something solid for support. The key is in pushing the hips back and the head forward to really stretch out the lower back.

Keep the body straight as you do so, no twisting in this movement!

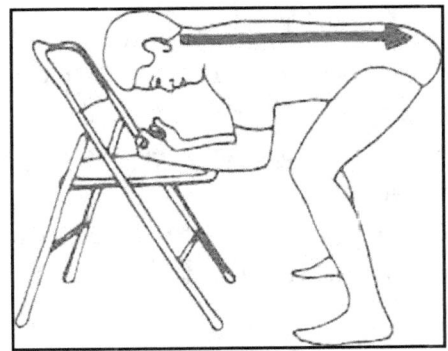

Two Hands Hold the Feet

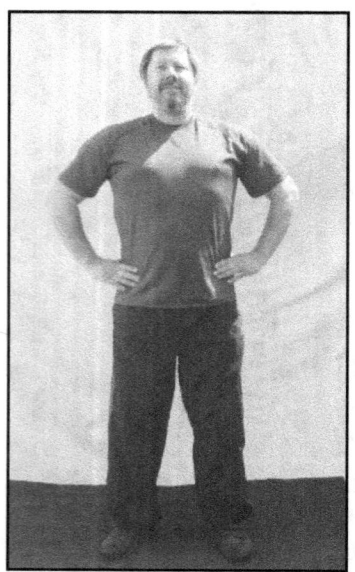 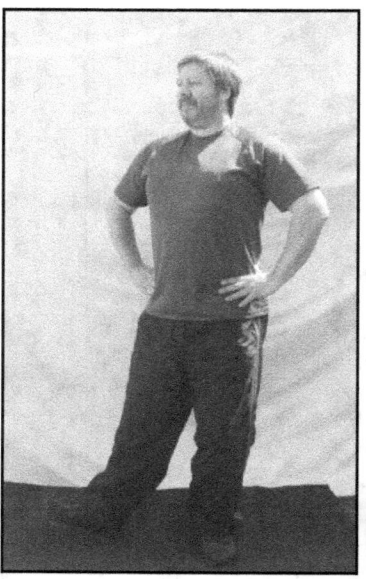 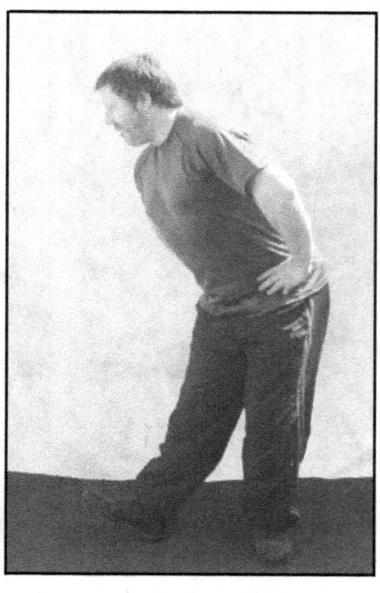

Stand in normal stance with hands on the hips. Start to inhale.

Shift the weight into the left leg. Turn to the right and raise the right toes.

Start an exhale and, keeping the weight in the back leg, begin to bend forward. Lead with the head.

This is a very common stretching move in Chinese martial arts. In fact, some traditional schools refused to take on a student until they could perform this stretch "chin to ankle!"

Of course, that is an extreme version of this movement, best started when you are very young!

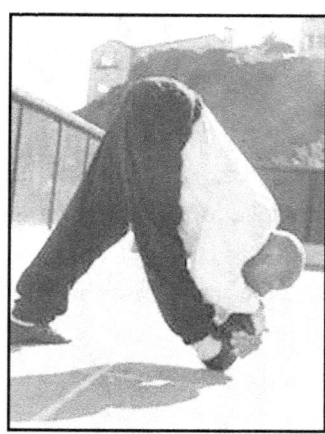

Simply Flow - The Eight Brocades

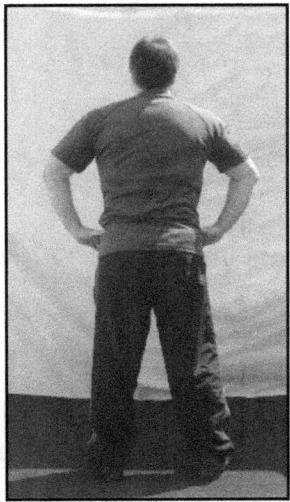
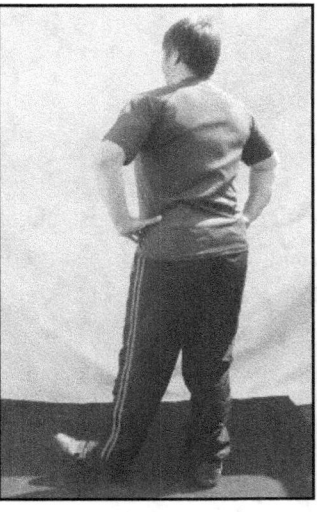
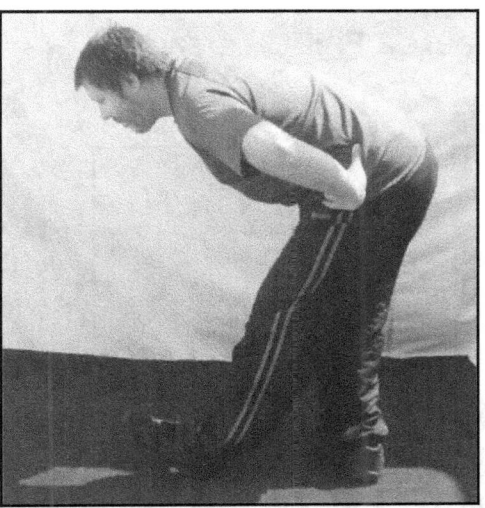

You can expand the chest on the inhale.

Always check your knee alignment, remember the foot and knee should point in the same direction.

When you bend be sure again to lead with the head and keep the lower back as straight as you can.

Just like the last exercise, you can also practice this movement as a static stretch.

Lean on something solid for support. The key again is in lengthening out the lower back and keeping the weight in the back leg.

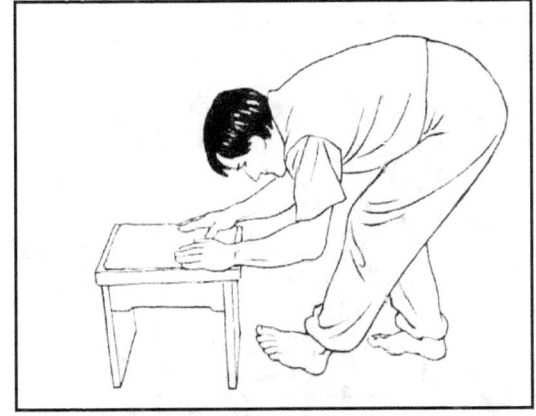

Seated Eight Brocades

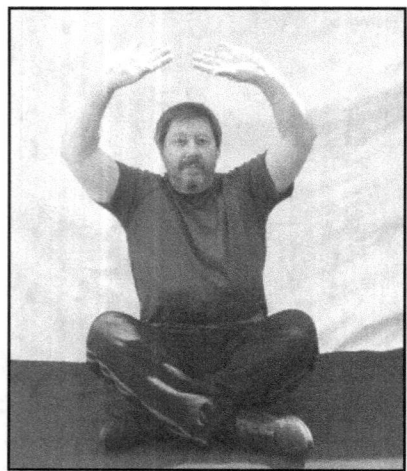

As we mentioned, it is possible to practice many of the Eight Brocades in a seated position. You can sit in a chair, or cross legged on the floor if you are comfortable in that position. The movements and breathing remain largely the same.

You can also still practice open and close in the hands and in the chest / back in the seated position

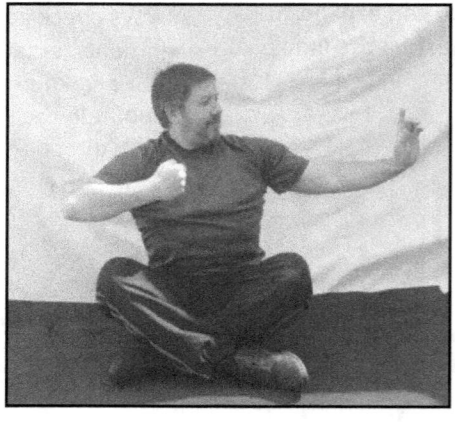

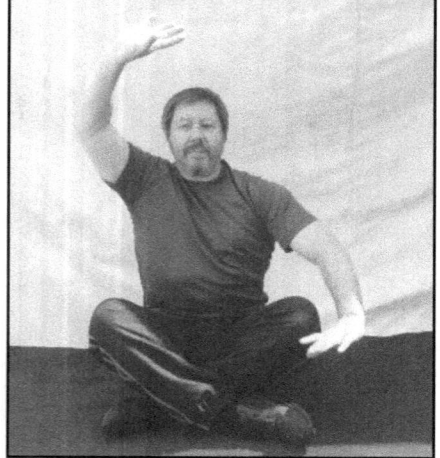

It may be more difficult to do some of the bending or twisting moves, though they may still be possible to some extent if you work from a chair.

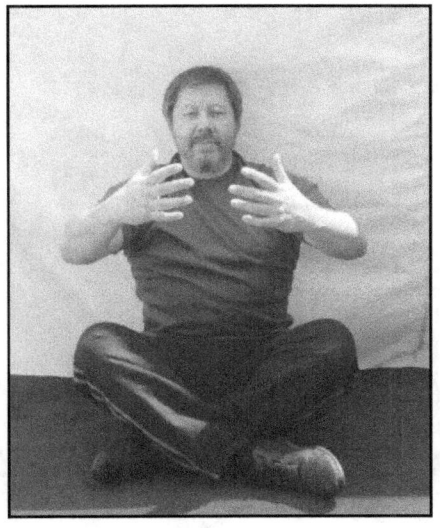 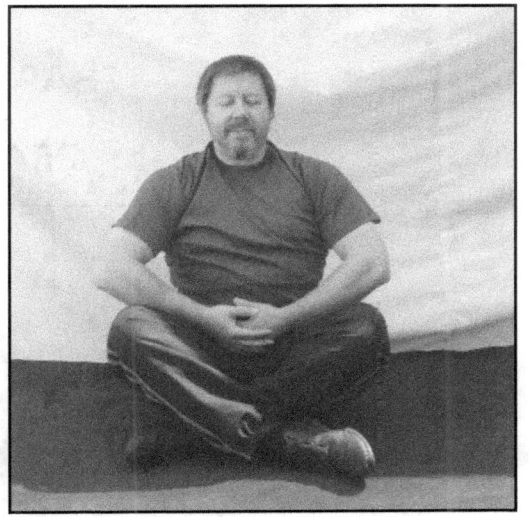

You can also practice Zhan Zhuang in the seated position. The arms are held in the *Holding the Jug* position to start.
When the arms lower, place the palms on the knees.

The Open and Closing exercises can also be practiced seated. Alternatively, you can just use the final resting position as a mediation posture. Remember to keep the back straight, no slouching!

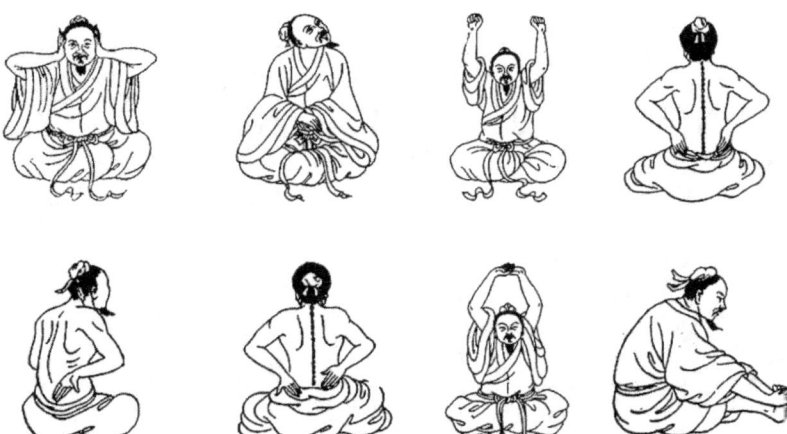

CHAPTER FIVE
PRACTICE

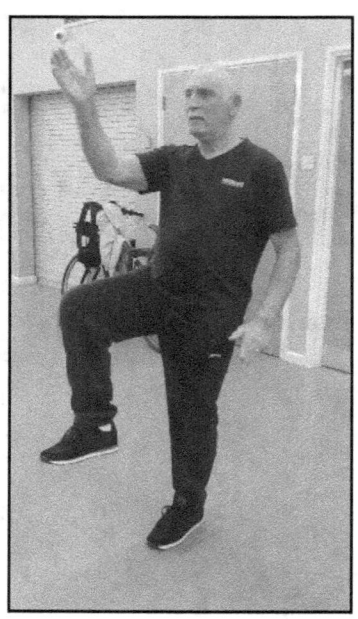

PRACTICE

So these are our Eight Brocade exercises, plus some variations. Again, I recommend you run through each exercise step by step. Start with a few repetitions of the basic movement, then you can start adding in all the other layers.

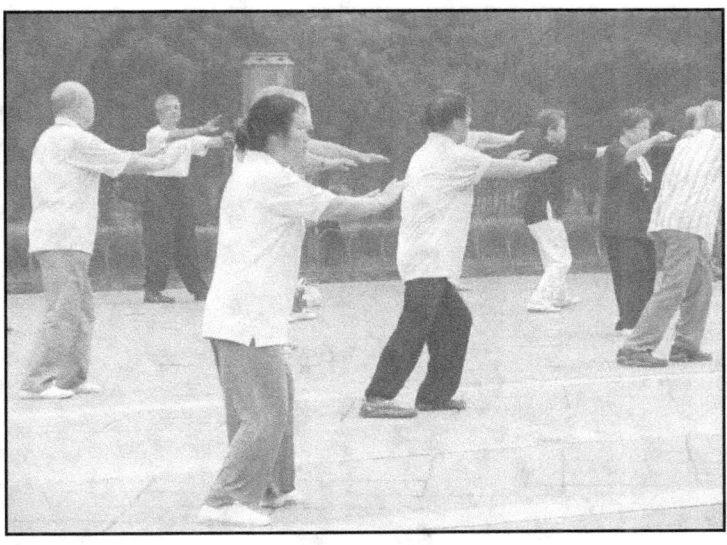

How much time you spend on the routine is up to you. You can run through a little breathing and perhaps two or three of the exercises if you don't have a lot of time. On the other hand, it's good practice to, say once a week, set aside an hour to run through all the breathing, Zhan Zhuang and a good number of reps of the whole routine.

The beauty of the Eight Brocades is that you can very easily fit it into your daily life. Taiji, for example, takes up quite a lot of space. Gym exercise may require special equipment and you may need a shower after. The Eight Brocades can be practiced pretty much on the spot. Furthermore, as we have seen, they can be adapted for different situations.

Something else to consider is just taking part of an exercise and practicing it as you need it. You may be sat at your computer all day, for example, and feel the need to stretch. Run through Two Hands Hold up the Heavens a few times. Or, while sitting, twist the body a few times to the left and right. This way you can often deal with tension before it has a chance to get a hold on you.

This is very much in line with the *Simply Flow* approach to health and fitness. We do not see exercise as something that is only practiced at set times, and is always "by the numbers". We see exercise as a natural part of our everyday lives. For this reason we prefer to often use the term *activity* rather than *exercise*! Because an activity is something you do all the time and is a natural part of your routine - such as brushing your teeth or taking the dog for a walk. If you can integrate all your exercise methods into your activities, you will start to discover a whole new layer of benefits to what can, otherwise, sometimes become a bit of a dull routine.

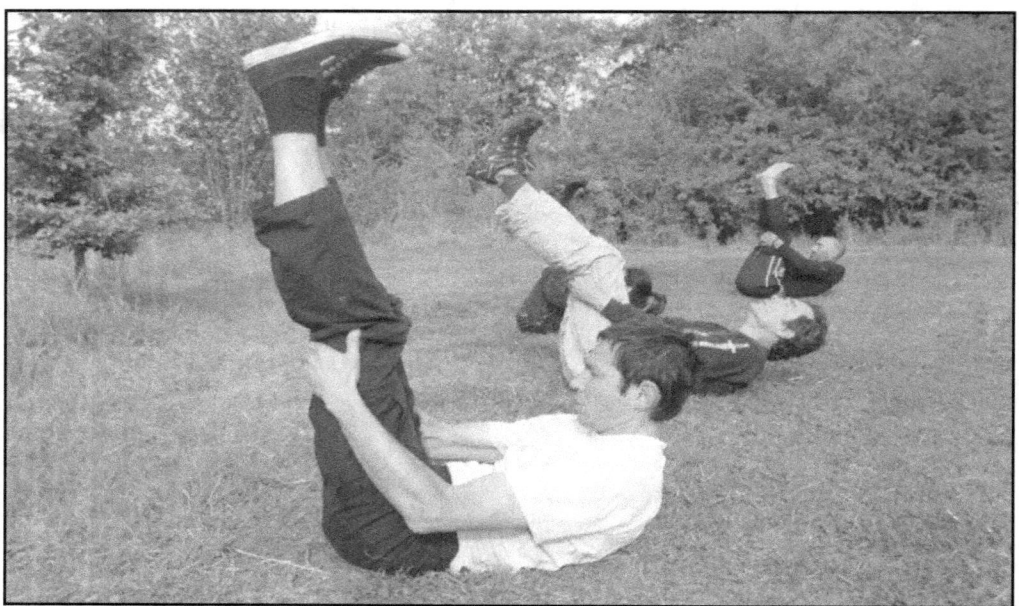

This goes double for the breathing! We have touched briefly on breath work in this book, but even this level of work can bring profound results. Get used to monitoring your breath throughout the day, particularly when you are getting stressed or tired. Quite often, in tense situations, we hold our breath, which does nothing but lock any tension into the muscles. If not addressed, that tension can seep deep into the muscle and cause problems later on.

Where to practice is another consideration. Traditionally, Qigong, Taiji and similar disciplines are practiced outdoors in the early morning, under trees is possible. These are said to be the optimum conditions to get maximum benefit from the exercises. It's a nice feeling to train outside, especially barefoot, if the ground surface allows it. It helps us to reconnect with nature. Don't be put off if the weather is not too good either. Training in the rain or cold can be very refreshing, as long as you are sensible. As the old saying goes, there's no such thing as bad weather, just the wrong type of clothing!

If you are outdoors, try and find a nice, private spot. You will by surprised at how even the most quiet place suddenly seems to attract activity as soon as you start meditation work! We have a running joke in one of our Taiji classes, which runs in a peaceful village gym.

So far we have had to contend with a low-flying Spitfire practicing aerobatics directly above us, a nearby neighbour deciding to angle-grind just after we started and all sorts of other

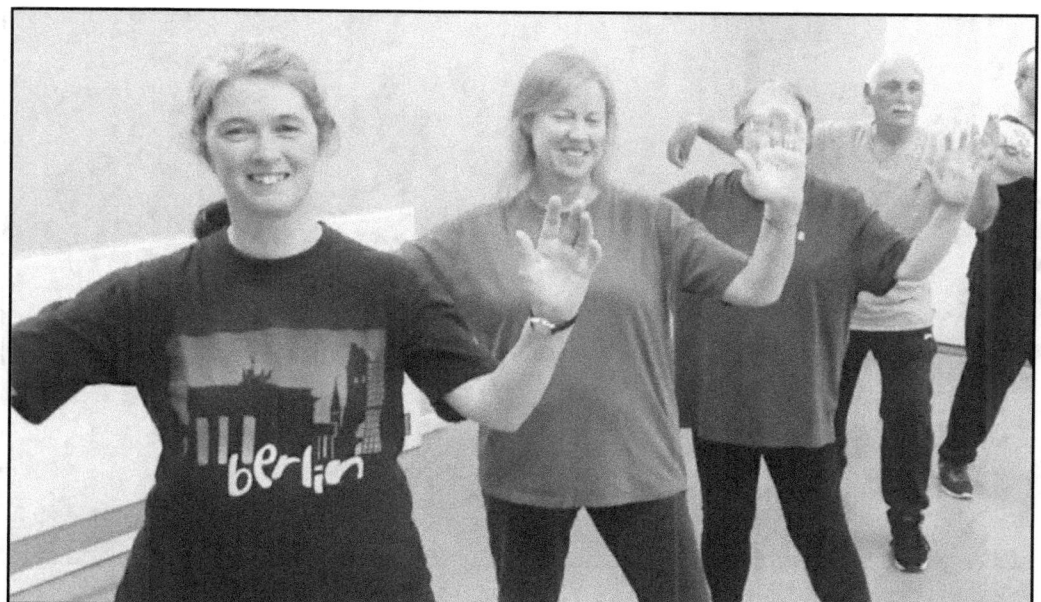

noises and distractions that seem to just be waiting for us to start our class! Now this can all be part of the challenge of finding "inner peace" but it is so much easier if you have a quiet place to start with. Meditation is a huge topic in itself but mindful movement, such as the Eight Brocades, is a very good starting point. Over time, you will develop the ability to carry that mindfulness over into your everyday activities, much the same as with the physical aspect of the exercises.

Of course, the Eight Brocades are only one form of exercise. There are many other aspects of health and fitness to explore. The best types enhance other activities. Qigong, for example, will help with posture and breathing for sports. There are plenty of exercises types that sit well alongside qigong. Stretching, pilates, various types of martial art, for example.

The main thing to consider with any form of exercise is the issue of safety and wear and tear, particularly as we get a bit older. There are some quite popular forms of training around that pay no attention to posture and body structure, place no emphasis on breathing and tend to load the body with more tension rather than releasing it. They can give people a quick "fitness buzz" and may develop good cardio but long term they can create problems..

Part of the difficulty is that when it comes to marketing, tension sells! Shaped muscles, fast movement, loud music, all have an appeal and give an impression of effective training. What the adverts fail to show are the long term costs of sustained, high-intensity training. There's a

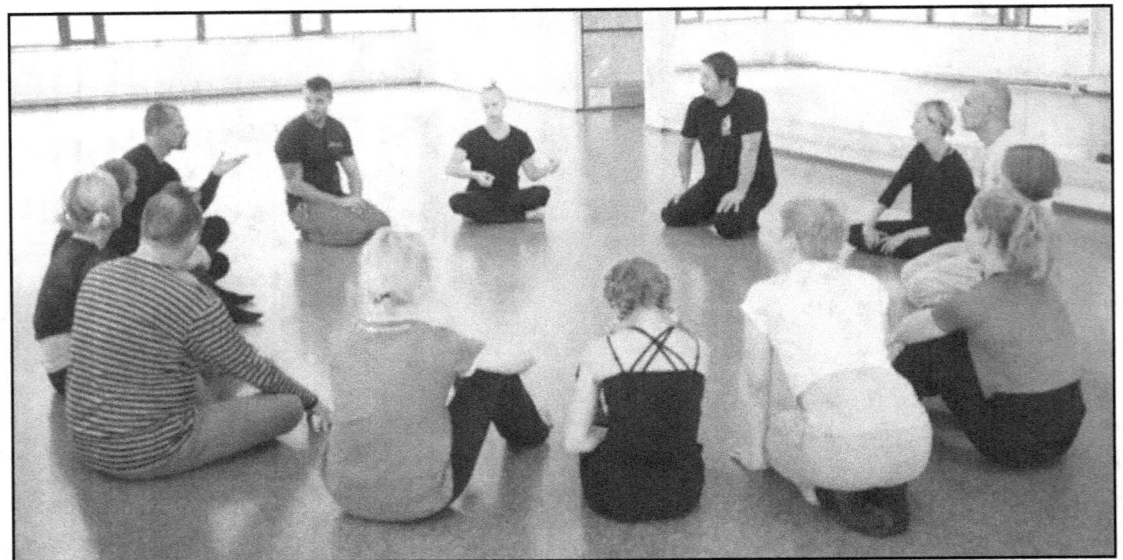

reason professional athletes have a relatively narrow career window!

So choose any form of exercise with care and do a little research! If you are going along to a class or session, never be afraid to ask an instructor questions. Sometimes it's also good to chat to the other people in the group to get their feedback on the training too. Over the years I've met and trained with many different teachers and some of the best ones were the least likely looking - so don't be taken in by snazzy outfits and slick marketing!

Speaking of groups, is it best to train qigong alone, or as part of a group? Each has its pros and cons. Working with a group can help in remembering the moves. It can also help with discipline - you have to exercise for the same amount of time as everyone else, so you can't be lazy!

You can also get a nice group atmosphere going, too. When everyone is breathing and moving in sync, it creates a very nice feeling in the training space.

The downside of group training is you have to find a time and a place convenient for everyone. In the Far East it is totally normal to see people, alone or in large groups, practicing qigong, Taiji and many other things in public parks. This is still quite a rare thing to see in the UK and you may find you attract attention. When we did early morning sessions in the local woods, the biggest problem was dogs out for a walk. they all wanted to come over and say "hello!"

Another thing when working with a group is you may feel obliged to always work at the

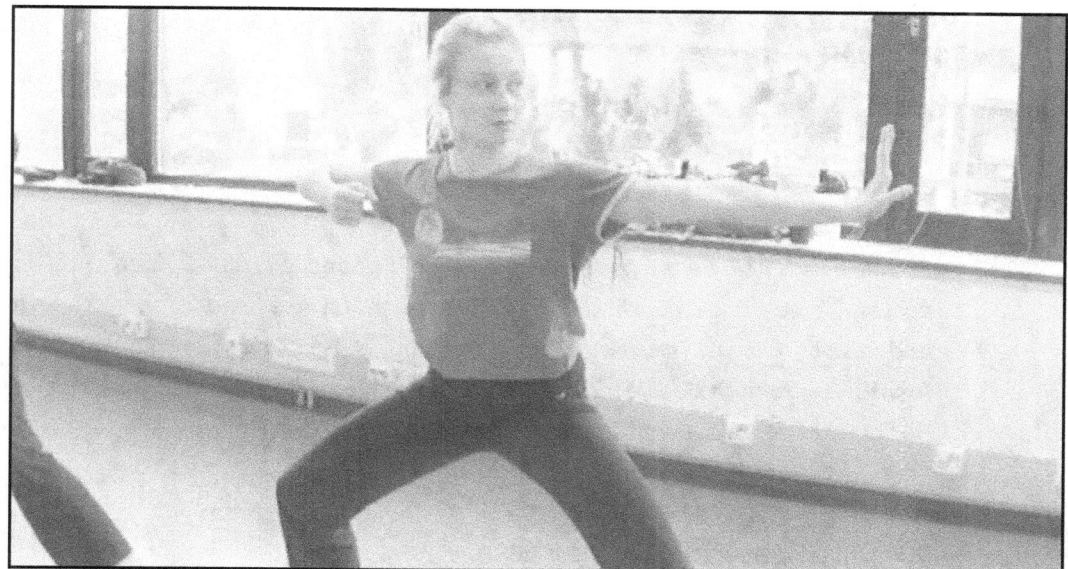

same speed as everyone else. This gives you less chance to work at your own speed. In my own classes I like to alternate. So sometimes we practice at "group speed" at other times I tell students to work at their own breathing rate. Both are equally valid and useful.

Working with a group and Instructor can also help with structuring your training. Having said that, the Eight Brocades are quite straightforward in terms of practice and progression. You may find, though, that some aspects, particularly the Silk Reeling methods, are easier to learn under the guidance of an experienced practitioner. Likewise, such a person can advise you on any issues you may be having, or suggest variations and enhancements of the basic movements.

However and wherever you choose to practice, I do hope you find benefit and enjoyment from practicing the Eight Brocades. They have been a part of my own personal training routine for decades now and I find there is always something new to learn! If you do have any questions or suggestions, or if you would like to find out more about *Simply Flow* classes, workshops and personal training, please do get in touch - the contact details are at the end of the book.

I wish you good health, a long and active life and happy training!

APPENDIX ONE

THE EIGHT BROCADE VERSES

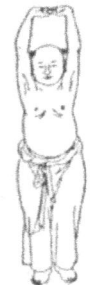

1. Two Hands Hold up the Heavens

Double hands hold up the heavens to regulate the Sanjiao (Triple Burner); Sanjiao passes Qi freely and smoothly, illnesses disappear. Reverse hands to face the sky and raise both arms. Thrust out (straighten) your chest, straighten your waist (and) swing to both sides. Stand upright and be steady. Practice long, the body (becomes) strong (and you will feel) happy.

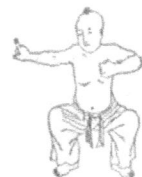

2. Pulling the Bow to Shoot the Hawk

Left right open (bend) the bow like shooting a hawk, two arms strong and firm to strengthen kidneys and waist. Bend the elbow horizontal to the shoulder, (your mind) trying hard to pull. Hand arrow aims (at the target), use the eyes to stare. Left right shoot for twenty-four. Ride the horse and squat down to increase efficiency.

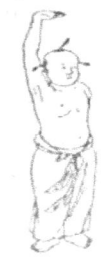

3. Separating Heaven And Earth

To adjust and regulate the spleen and stomach, (you) must lift singly; spleen and stomach (gain) peace and harmony, sickness cured automatically. Lift arm and stiffen the palms, use the force to rock. Extend and develop the tendons and muscles, spleen and stomach comfortable. Right hand lifted high, left dropped down, left right extend and rock the tendons and channels alive.

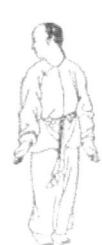

4. Turn and Gaze at the Moon

Five weaknesses and seven injuries, wait and see later (they'll be gone); train long, exercise long, tendons and bones strong. Weakness injuries (from over exertion) all because the internal organs (are) weak. Thrust out (straighten) the chest and twist the neck to take a good look to the rear. Hold the waist and hold up the chest; the body is upright. This is especially effective in curing internal injury.

5. Sway Head and Swing Tail

Sway the head and swing the tail to get rid of the heart fire. (When) the heart fire (is) strong, (use) the metal lung to subdue. Hands press the kneecaps,-repeatedly sway and swing. Blood flows smoothly, many good benefits. (If) the muscles and tendons are cramped, legs sore, (and) body numb, repeatedly extend and press heavily; do not waste time (hesitate).

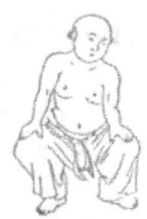

6. Two Hands Hold the Feet

Two hands hold the feet to strengthen the kidneys and waist; (when the) kidneys and waist are strong the entire body (is) strong. Bend the waist and hold the feet. (This is the) most effective way to strengthen the muscles/tendons and bones. One down one up, the life force greatly increases. (It is) the best way to prevent colds

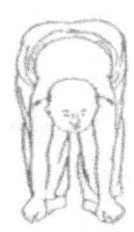

7. Clench the Fists and Glare Fiercely

Screw the fist with fiery eyes to increase qi-li; body and mind healthy, the spirit of vitality comfortable. Ride the horse and squat down, straightening the chest. Hold the fist or strike with palm, using more force. Left and right, two hands grasp in turn. Grasp, hold, fiery eyes, use li-qi.

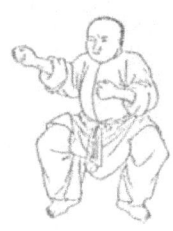

8. Bouncing on the Toes

Seven disorders and hundreds of illnesses disappear and are left behind your back; hundreds of illnesses are caused because the body is weak. The feet up, achievement is hard to describe by pen. Keep the head up and press down to reach to the end of the toes. Hold the waist and hold the chest, up and down movements. (It is) effective in getting rid of sickness and eliminating disasters (illnesses).

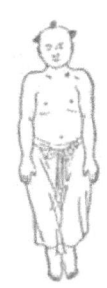

APPENDIX TWO

MERIDIAN CHARTS

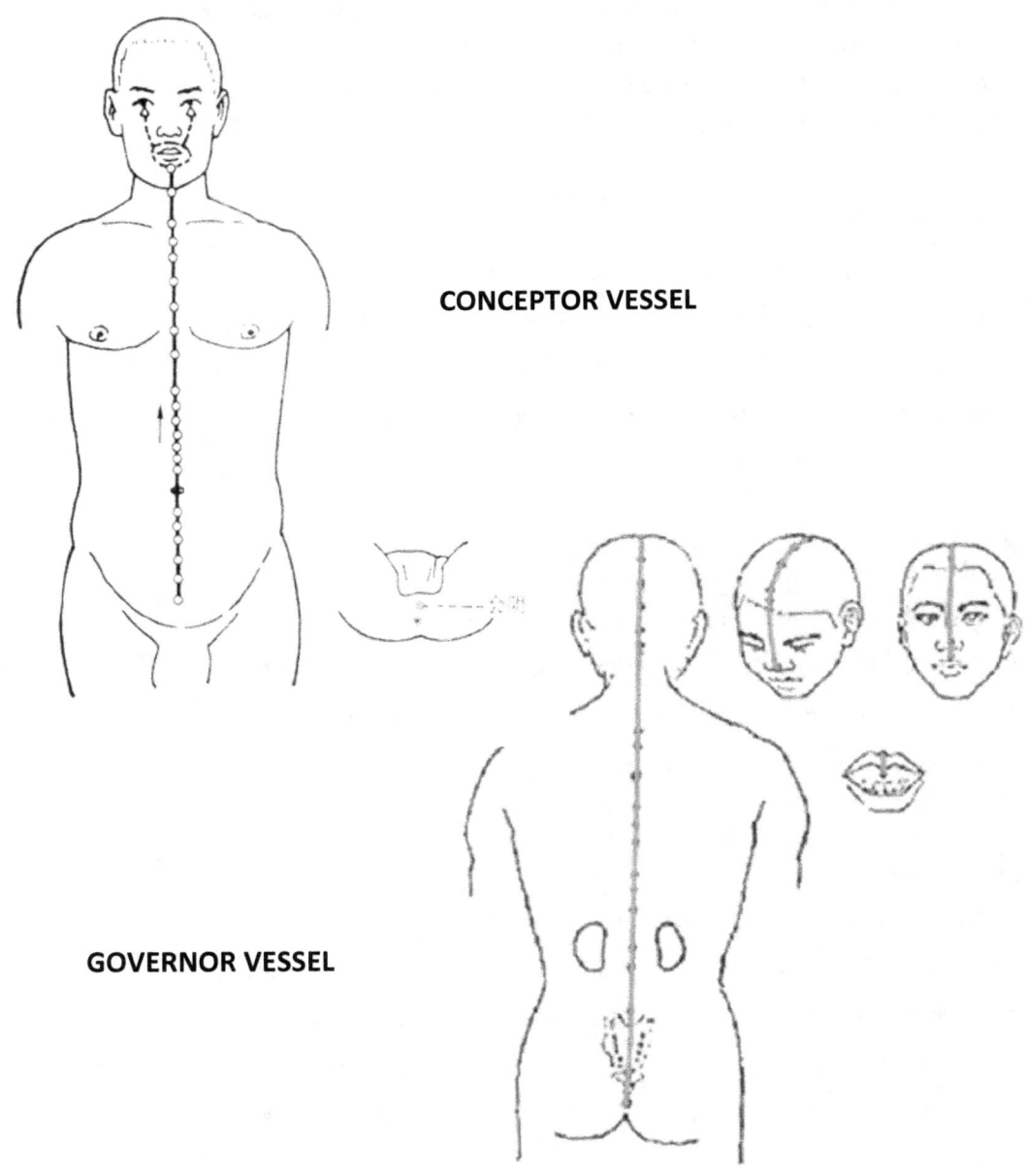

CONCEPTOR VESSEL

GOVERNOR VESSEL

KIDNEY MERIDIAN

LARGE INTESTINE MERIDIAN

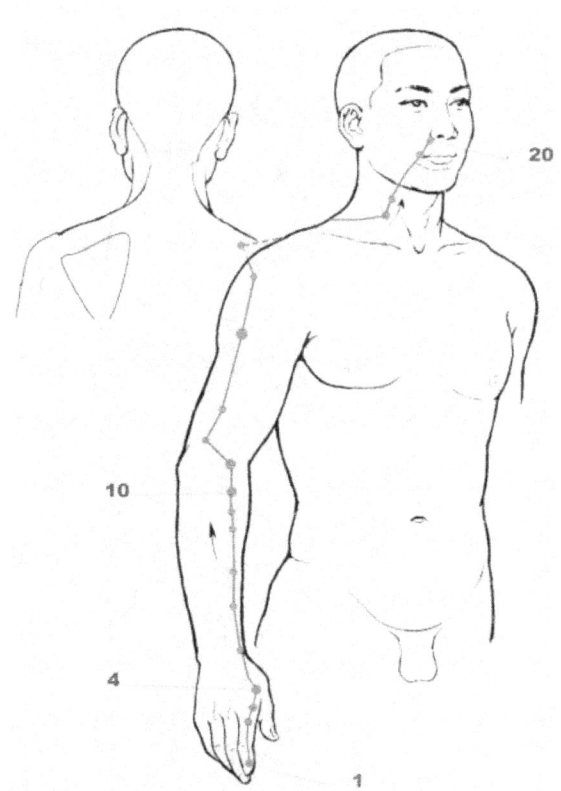
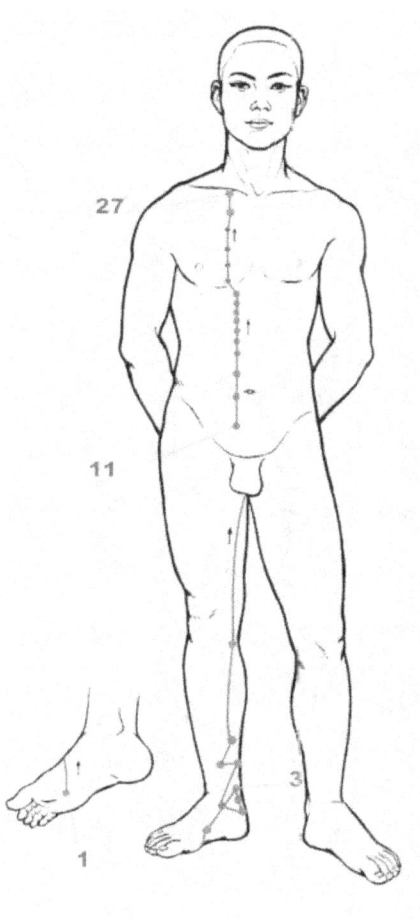

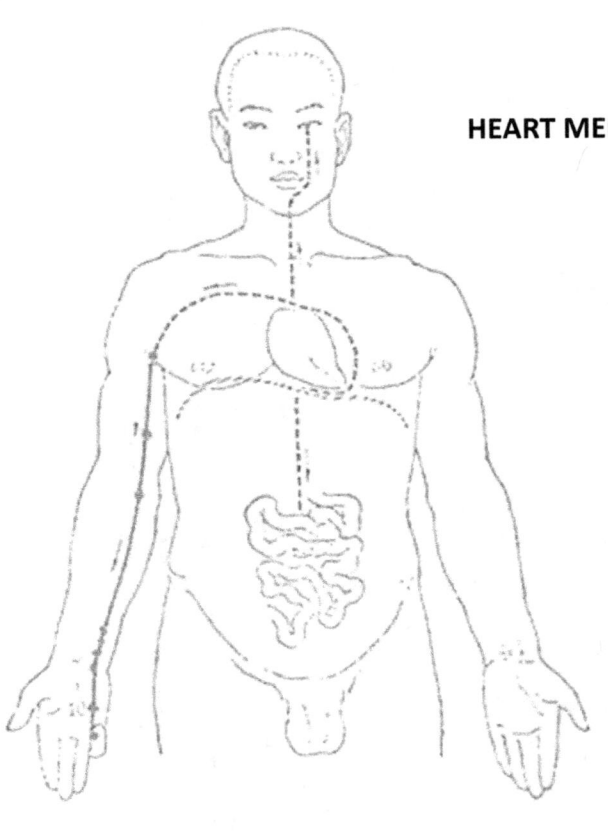

HEART MERIDIAN

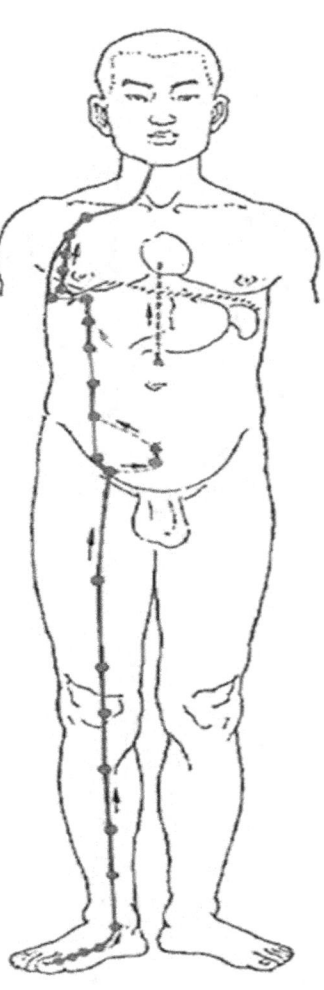

SPLEEN MERIDIAN

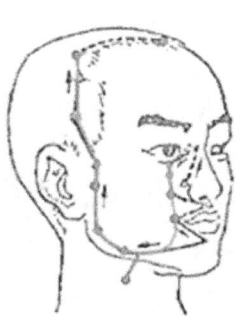
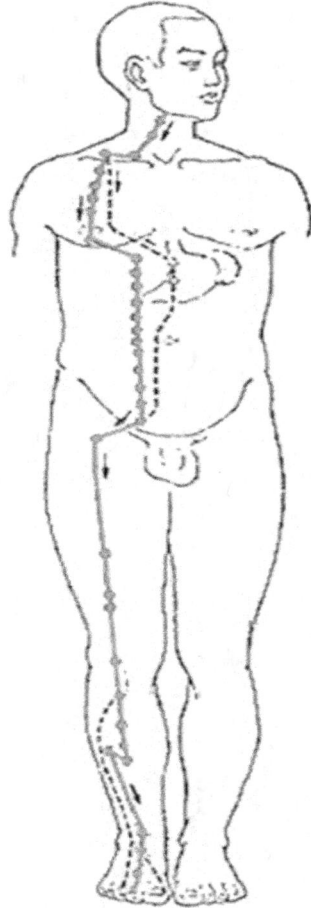

STOMACH MERIDIAN

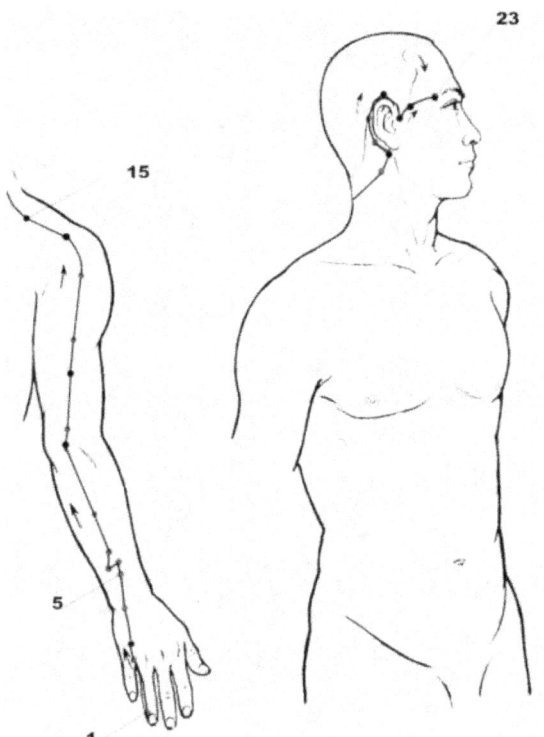

TRIPLE WARMER MERIDIAN

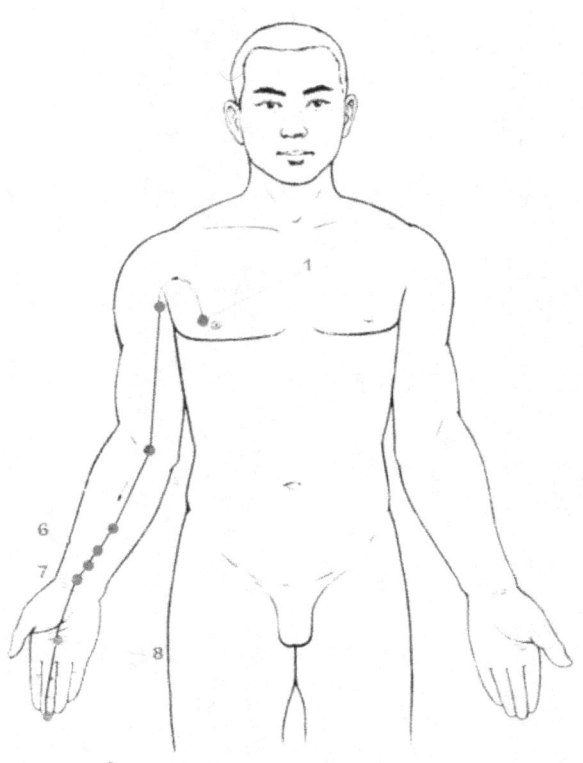

PERICARDIUM MERIDIAN

LUNG MERIDIAN

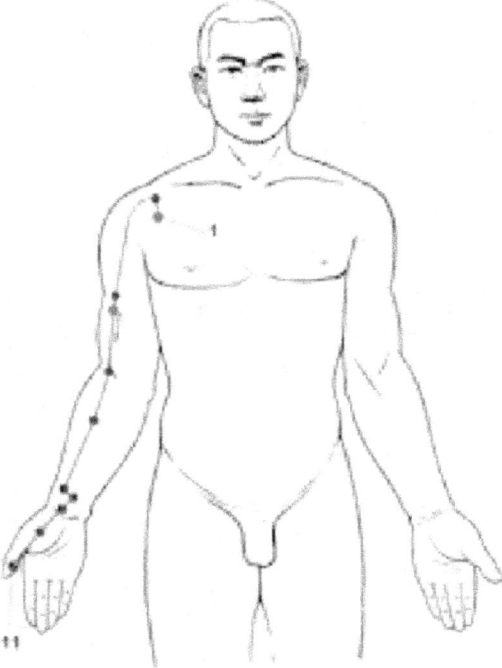

SMALL INTESTINE MERIDIAN

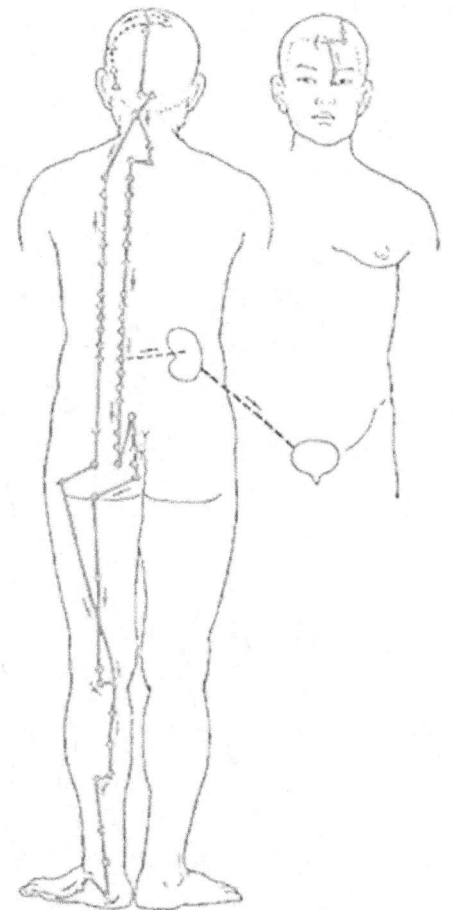

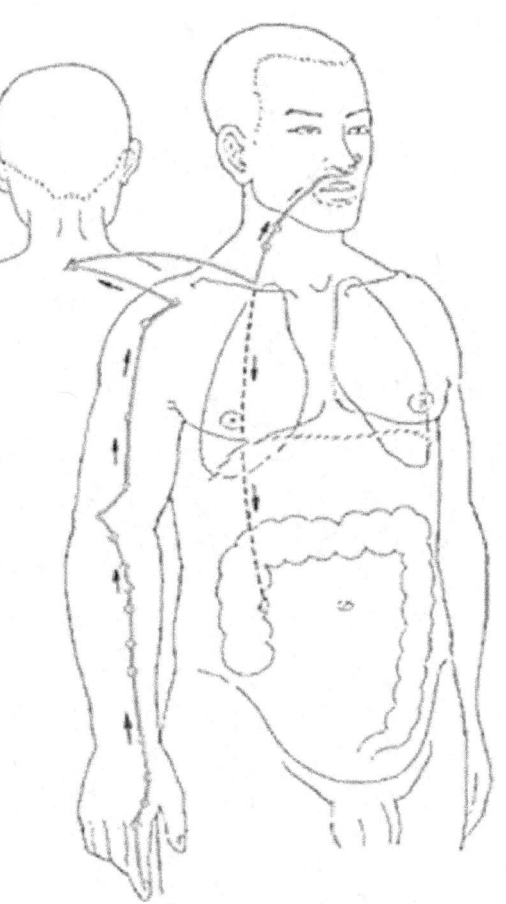

BLADDER MERIDIAN

LIVER MERIDIAN

GALL BLADDER MERIDIAN

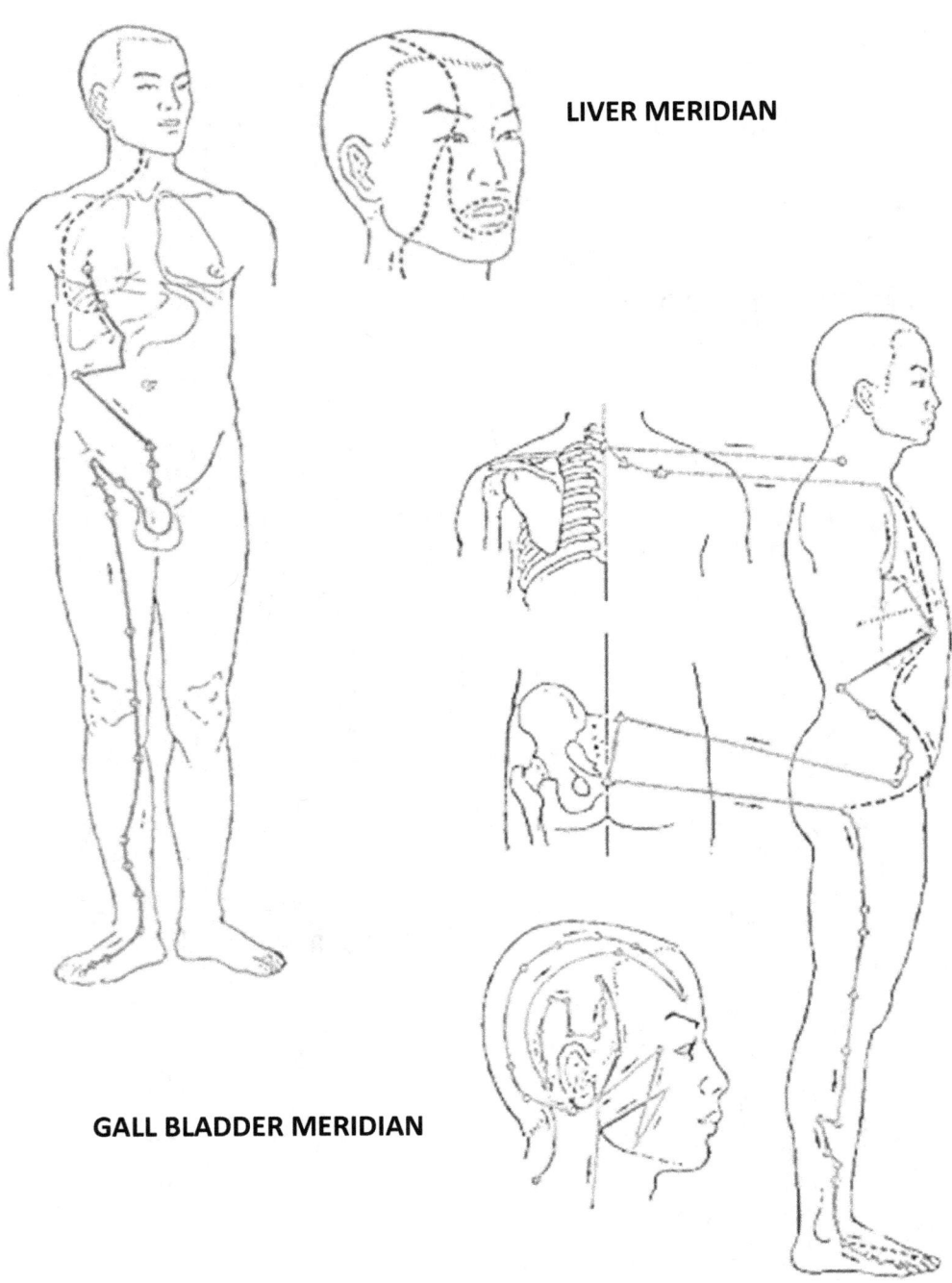

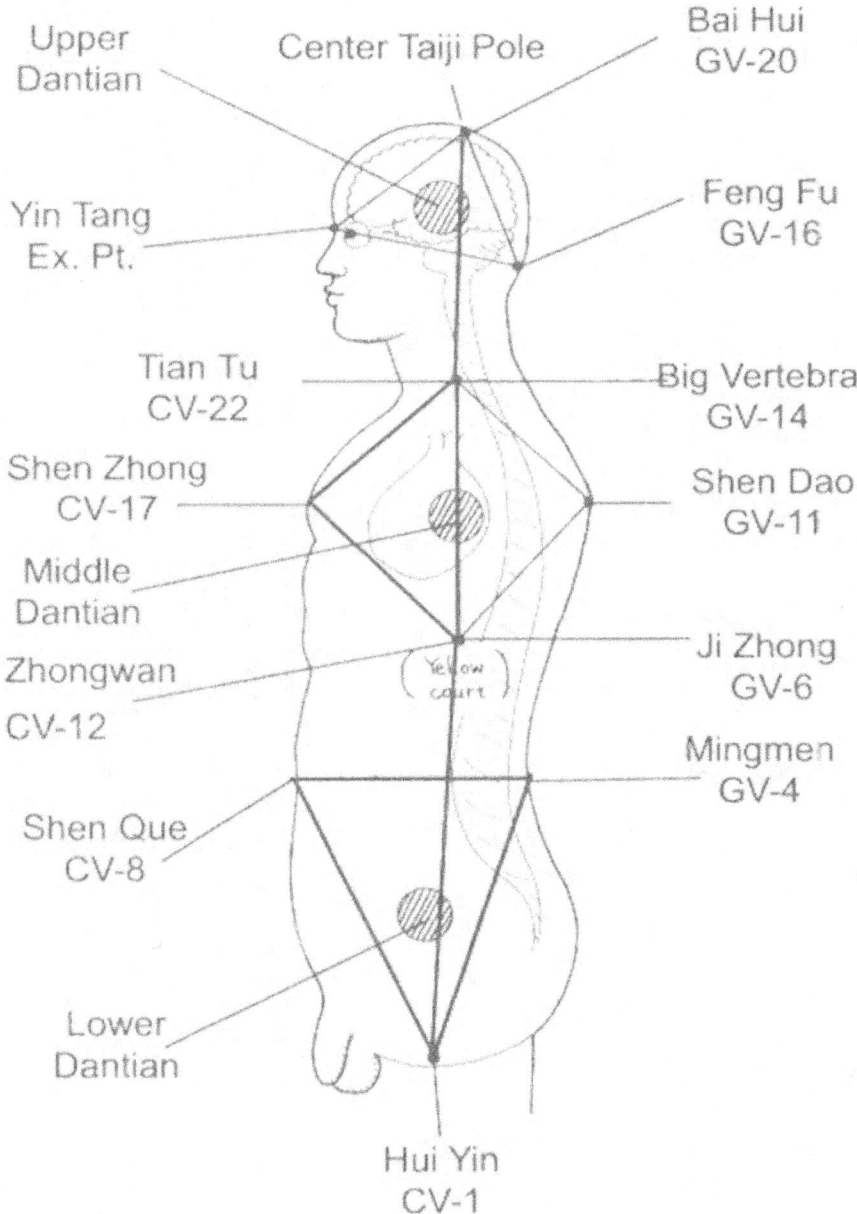

APPENDIX THREE

CONTACT DETAILS

    E-MAIL   simplyflow@outlook.com

    WEBSITE   www.simplyflow.co.uk

    FACEBOOK GROUP   www.facebook.com/simplyflowgroup/

    SHOP SITE   www.systemafilms.com

Sign up to our mailing list for news and offers! http://eepurl.com/dmNQhz

If you have enjoyed this book, please leave us a review on Amazon.
Thanks!

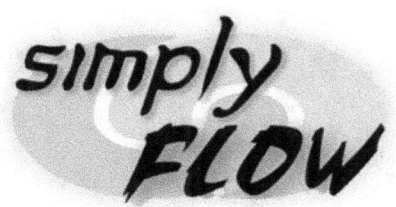

NOTES

NOTES

Simply Flow - The Eight Brocades

ALSO AVAILABLE FROM SIMPLY FLOW!

FITNESS OVER 40

Many people ask how they can maintain health and fitness as they age. Gyms can be expensive and intimidating and many exercise programs focus solely on superficial looks.

The *Simply Flow* Program is all about regaining your body's natural movement, building core strength, boosting your health and learning to manage stress and tension.

It involves simple to learn exercises that easily fit into and enhance all your other activities, as well as giving you a unique Formula to develop your own exercise variations. This book covers all the foundation exercises of the Program, including -

Breathing
Core Strength
Joint Mobility
Stretching
Movement Chains
Resistance Training
Ground Movement
Mindfulness and Flow

Plus advice on diet, lifestyle, developing your own training routines and more.

Looking for a sensible long term exercise program that fits in with and enhances your lifestyle and activities?

Here it is!

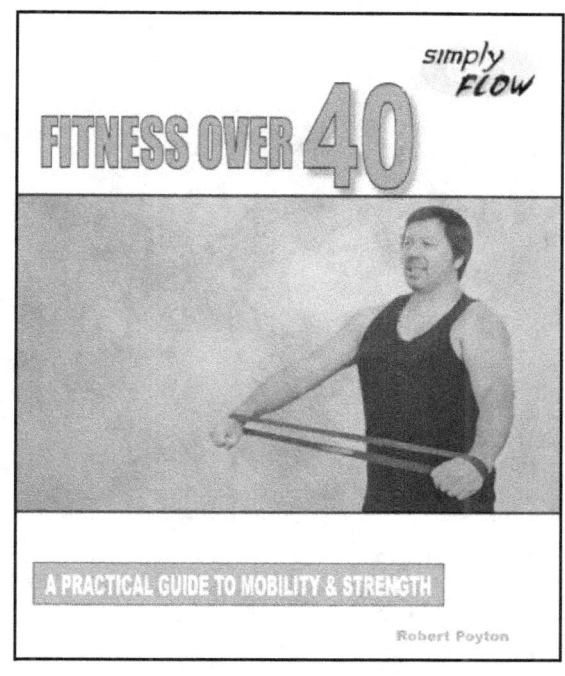

Large paperback 126 pages
Fully illustrated
Available via Amazon or direct from

www.simplyflow.co.uk

www.ingramcontent.com/pod-product-compliance
Lightning Source LLC
Chambersburg PA
CBHW051420070526
44584CB00023B/3506